AIDS,
The
Winter
War

AIDS,
The
Winter
War

• • •

ARTHUR D. KAHN

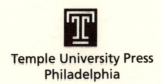

Temple University Press
Philadelphia

Temple University Press, Philadelphia, PA 19122

∞ The paper used in this publication meets the minimum requirements of American National Standard for Information Sciences—Permanence of Paper for Printed Library Materials, ANSI Z39.48–1984

Printed in the United States of America

Library of Congress Cataloging-in-Publication Data

Kahn, Arthur David.
    AIDS, the winter war / Arthur D. Kahn.
      p.   cm.
    Includes index.
    ISBN 1–56639–018–4
    1. AIDS (Disease)—United States. 2. Pharmaceutical policy—United States. 3. AIDS (Disease)—Government policy—United States. I. Title.
RA644.A25K34 1992 1993
362.1'969792'00973—dc20   92–15423

These are the times that try men's souls. The summer soldier and the sunshine patriot will, in this crisis, shrink from the service of their country, but he that stands it now deserves the love and thanks of man and woman.

Tom Paine, *The Crisis*, 1776

CONTENTS

◆ ◆ ◆

PART II

PREFACE

◆ ◆ ◆

The origin of this book dates back to the fall of 1985.

"An Early Frost" provided the impulse—a television play about a young man dying of AIDS who is rejected by his parents when they learn for the first time of his homosexuality.

As the play progressed, I was overcome both with sorrow at the suffering of the afflicted and with shame at my inaction. Having undergone open-heart surgery a few months earlier, I was limited in what I could do, but I had time to spare. A retired professor, my days were my own. Only proofreading of galleys remained with a book on which I had been working for the previous twelve years. That book, *The Education of Julius Caesar*, would be brought out first as the History Book Club selection of July 1986 and formally published by Schocken Books two months later.

The next morning I called the Gay Men's Health Crisis (GMHC), and for several months at the headquarters I stuffed envelopes, typed, ran errands and took turns at the reception desk. I frequently was paired with a slight, bespectacled man in his early forties—cheerful, efficient, a volunteer almost every day. Once, when I had failed to see him for a week or so, I asked him whether he had been ill. "Often," he replied, "you see, I'm a PWA [Person with AIDS]." During a longer absence I discovered he was in the hospital with an eye infection, an opportunistic disease that often occurs with AIDS. I called. He was partly blind, he said, but hopeful of leaving the hospital soon. He died some days later.

On Tuesday evenings I volunteered at weekly dinners at St. Peter's Church in midtown Manhattan. Here I saw emaciated PWAs who resembled the liberated concentration-camp inmates I had seen in Germany at the end of World War II. Some of them were alone and broken in spirit and grateful for a smile or a stroke of affection. Others, more fortunate, were nursed by lovers, who supported them as they walked into the dining area and then sat with an arm about their shoulders.

At a Thanksgiving dinner for PWAs at the Episcopal church of St. John's in Greenwich Village, the priest asked everyone to state in turn what he or she was thankful for that afternoon. One man said, "Thanksgiving was always my favorite holiday. I looked forward to going home and being with my parents and my brothers and sisters. This year they would not have me because of my AIDS. I'm thankful that I have a family here."

I enrolled in a two-weekend GMHC training program, and for several months thereafter I worked with a "buddy" group in Brooklyn.

In February 1987 I attended a meeting at which Michael May, the director of a chorus in New Jersey, recounted how a year earlier, terminally ill with AIDS, he had traveled to Israel, undergone treatment with a variant of egg lecithin called AL721 and quickly regained his health and strength. When he reported that the Israelis would not accept any more American AIDS patients and refused to provide any explanation for this change in policy, he evoked an uproar of indignation in the audience.

I resolved to travel to Israel to investigate both the treatment itself and the reason for the refusal to accept additional American patients. Richard Dunne, director of GMHC, and Drs. Joseph Sonnabend and Mathilde Krim, two scientists who founded the American Foundation for AIDS Research, encouraged me in this project.

I would have left for Israel in June 1987 without adequate preparation if I had not had the assistance of John S. James. A Harvard graduate, John had worked as a data processor for the National Institutes of Health, taught in a community college and then held varied positions as a computer programmer. In 1986 he began writing a column for the San Francisco gay publication *The Sentinel* and joined the staff of a public service organization called the Documentation of AIDS Issues and Research Foundation (D.A.I.R.). Eventually, he established the *AIDS Treatment News*, an authoritative biweekly report on AIDS therapies in which he investigated new therapies and provided his readers with the history, the operating theory, the results of experiments and directions for making or obtaining substances. His publication became a clearinghouse of information for the AIDS community.

"I shouldn't be doing this work," John says of his newsletter. "It should have been started by the government years ago, but either I do it or it doesn't get done."

Upon learning of my intention to go to Israel to investigate AL721, John James telephoned to urge me to expand my research into a comprehensive study of the general problems in the development of new AIDS therapies. "You are the first person," said John with enthusiasm, "whom I have been able to persuade to undertake such a project."

At the Weizmann Institute in Israel, the scientist responsible for the development of AL721, Meir Shinitzky, a guileless and affable individual, welcomed me without any questions as to my motives or my qualifications. I disarmed his suspicious associate David Samuel by noting with humor that having met not only viscounts but even marquesses while a liaison officer at Montgomery's headquarters during the Battle of the Bulge in World War II, I was not intimidated by his title (he is Viscount Samuel). I further reassured him by observing that one of my purposes in writing a book was to give the Israelis deserved credit for the development of a therapy that offered promise for the treatment not only of AIDS but of other disorders as well. I spoke at length also with three Israeli physicians who were treating AIDS patients with AL721.

From Israel I traveled to France, where at Clermont-Ferrand a physician whom I had met during World War II arranged an appointment for me with scientists who had experimented with AL721 with cystic fibrosis patients.

In London Dr. Anthony Pinching, a scientist who was planning to conduct a clinical trial of AL721, was just leaving for Kenya. I had an opportunity, however, to discuss my experiences in Israel with members of the Terrence Higgins Foundation, the London counterpart to New York's GMHC. I corresponded with Dr. Pinching after returning to New York.

Michael May's "recovery" through the Israeli therapy, publicized widely in the media, along with the simultaneous federal authorization of the compound AZT, evoked a change in atmosphere in the AIDS community and ushered in a new phase in the swiftly evolving history of the epidemic. It was about this new phase that I planned to write a book.

Upon John James's inserting a notice in his *AIDS Treatment News* that I was seeking information for a book about AL721, I began receiving calls from all over the country from individuals either eager to recount their personal experience or seeking information about the therapy. Among the callers was Linda Hunt, the public relations director for Ethigen,[1] the company authorized by the Israelis for world distribution of AL721.[2] She proposed a collaboration. After I set as a condition that there be no waffling on even embarrassing questions, I had no further communication with Ms. Hunt. My telephone messages were ignored, and scientists engaged on company projects refused to talk to me.

I began an intensive schedule of interviews, speaking with scientists who had done research on AL721, with physicians who had used it in treating patients, with leaders of activist organizations, with directors of groups distributing "underground" AIDS therapies and with PWAs using the substance. In July I established contact with the Washington law firm conducting a class action suit launched by the National Gay Rights Advocates against the Department of Health and Human Services and its dependent public health agencies on the charge of procrastination in the release of AIDS therapies. Two members of the firm came to New York and spent three hours taping me on my findings regarding AL721. Thereafter we continued to exchange information.

---

[1] In May 1987 the name of the firm was changed from Praxis to Ethigen.

[2] There are variations in the spelling of the egg lecithin variant. Except in quoted passages, I have used the Israeli spelling.

Another source for information, efficiently organized and geared for immediate response, was the Documentation of AIDS Issues and Research Foundation. Donald J. Gorman, 36, founded the organization and served as its president until August 1987, when he was diagnosed with AIDS. He and Michael Flanagan, the subsequent president, and Ken McPherson, a coordinator of the Mobilization Against AIDS, periodically issued the "D.A.I.R. Update," a ten-page condensation of important news about AIDS. In addition, they filed and cataloged research materials for the use of reporters, researchers and others interested in the AIDS problem. Project Inform, another San Francisco AIDS information organization, also proved a useful source. I came to rely considerably for information and advice upon the co-director, Martin Delaney, one of the most knowledgeable individuals in the United States on all aspects of the AIDS struggle. In the fall of 1987 Dr. Barry Gingell, medical consultant for the GMHC, and Kevin Armington began publishing *Treatment Issues*, a GMHC newsletter of experimental AIDS therapies and an invaluable source of carefully researched investigations.

In February 1987, when I first learned about AL721, I was not aware of the establishment of the PWA Health Group, an organization planning to distribute the egg lecithin variant developed by the Israelis. During the spring and summer of 1987 similar distribution groups were formed in numerous cities throughout the country as well as in other countries. The organization of these groups signaled a new stage in the AIDS crisis: the stage of PWA self-empowerment.

Another aspect of the story of AL721 was the role of the activists who organized protests to prod governmental agencies and of those individuals outside official agencies who carried on research projects, assembled data and publicized new developments in the confrontation with the epidemic.

Their story deserved recounting.

As I pursued my investigations during the last months of 1987, I became ever more aware that I would have to set the investigation of AL721 within a broad context, exploring, for example, the roles of the Food and Drug Administration (FDA) and of the National Institutes of Health (NIH) in the testing and authorization of AL721. I would also have to compare their handling of AL721 with their handling of other potential AIDS therapies.[3] (I offer no personal judgment regarding AL721, which by 1990 generally was rejected as an AIDS therapy although numerous PWAs as well as Israeli physicians continued to use it.)

The first half of this book describes the reawakening of gay militancy following

---

[3] A retired Classics professor, I have no pretensions to medical knowledge more recent than the writings of Hippocrates. I can offer no judgment regarding the efficacy of AL721 in the treatment of AIDS. At the time of the writing of this book, no decisive large-scale, multicenter clinical trials of the substance had been completed. On the other hand, in January 1988, after experiencing a distressing decline in energy because of my cardiac condition, following advice at the Weizmann Institute, where the original investigations with AL721 had been conducted with geriatric patients, I began taking a small daily dose of the egg lecithin variant. Within about three months my energy returned, and my cardiologist, surprised at the change in my condition, permitted me to renew my working out with Nautilus machines.

the realization by the AIDS community that because of the failure of government at various levels to confront the epidemic expeditiously, the community would have to mount ever more vigorous pressure to expose official neglect and dawdling. In addition, AIDS activists would have to keep watch on pharmaceutical corporations exploiting the crisis for quick and often exorbitant profits rather than out of a sense of public service. To this end the activists would have to gain sophistication regarding the procedures and personalities in FDA, the Centers for Disease Control (CDC) and NIH. They would have to become sufficiently informed about the virus to discuss meaningfully the direction and quality of HIV research and to distinguish the relative potential effectiveness of proposed therapies.

The rapidity and breadth of this preparation among AIDS activists will remain one of the wondrous achievements of the AIDS community during the period covered in this book. By the summer of 1987, when a new stage was inaugurated in the AIDS struggle through the appointment of the Presidential Commission on the Human Immunodeficiency Virus (HIV) Epidemic, AIDS activists were prepared to provide testimony on par with, and often superior to, that of professional expert witnesses.

Appointed in the summer of 1987 by a president who had consistently held to a do-nothing policy in face of an epidemic expanding in a geometrical progression that threatened the already weakened national health service, an economy weighed down by debts unprecedented in the nation's history and, indeed, of a disintegration of the fabric of the society—the Presidential Commission was greeted by the media, by the scientific and medical communities and especially by AIDS activists with cynicism and scorn.

To general astonishment, however, under the leadership of a retired admiral and former Chief of Naval Operations with no scientific or medical experience, the conservative Commissioners not only underwent an educational process comparable in swiftness to that among AIDS activists but ended their tenure with a Final Report that encompassed nearly all the demands that AIDS activists had been posing. Furthermore, as a result of the Commission's comprehensive investigation, far more ambitious than the AIDS community was capable of undertaking, the broad ramifications of the crisis were exposed. After the publication of the Final Report, no programs proposed for combating the epidemic could ignore such general questions as the state of national health services, the effectiveness of the war on drugs or the threat arising from an unrestricted emphasis on profit to the exclusion of concern for the general welfare as well as from an entire syndrome of social problems.

Admittedly, the division within this book—a first part on the self-education of AIDS activists and a second part on the education of the Commissioners during an intensive series of hearings on various aspects of the epidemic—may strike the reader as brusque. But developments traced in Part I continue and in some instances overlap developments presented in Part II.

In fact, however, the evolution of the AIDS community in intense, multifaceted struggles following swiftly one upon another culminates in the very special contribution of AIDS activists to the education of the Commissioners and thus to the drafting of the Commission's Final Report. Furthermore, with all due respect to his impressive leadership, the Commission's chairman, whether consciously or not, took his cues from the issues raised by the AIDS community and achieved his successes within the Commission because of a general environment and atmosphere set by the AIDS activists in their public demonstrations, in their remonstrances to government officials and agencies and in such self-defense operations as the establishment of AIDS service organizations and therapy distribution centers.

During the spring and summer of 1988 I interviewed three of the Commission's staff as well as four Commissioners, including the Commission chairman. In addition, during several days at Commission headquarters, I examined the voluminous transcripts of the Commission's hearings. With the publication in June of the Final Report, the nation possessed at last, after seven years of crisis and of federal neglect, a comprehensive program and a clearly defined direction for confronting the epidemic. Thereafter the struggle of the AIDS community was to be directed more and more toward the implementation of the proposals in this report, including proposals encompassing aspects of the struggle previously ignored or only superficially touched upon by AIDS activists.

Thus from a limited investigation of a promising AIDS therapy, this book evolved over the period of a year and a half to include an account of the struggle of the AIDS community against government inertia and, finally, into an investigation of the potentially catastrophic impact of the AIDS crisis on American society.

Over the many months of its composition this book evolved into a history of the AIDS struggle during two critical years. For such a book the present title is appropriate—*AIDS, The Winter War*.

Inspired by reading the manuscript to renew his AIDS research, Bill Regelson of the Medical College of Virginia, a distinguished scientist of broad medical interests, volunteered to write an introduction in which he would set in perspective the contribution of AIDS activists not merely in the struggle for people with HIV infection but for patients with other major diseases.

This is not my book. I serve merely as a chronicler. I have recounted the evolution of a group of privileged citizens appointed by a reactionary president indifferent to the AIDS crisis from what in practical effect represented obtuse ignorance to an awareness not only of the import of the epidemic for the future of the nation but also of new insights into the broad crisis of our society. Above all, I have sought to memorialize the heroic individuals, primarily PWAs, who mounted a struggle not only in defense of their own lives but also in pursuit of a truly kinder and gentler America.

INTRODUCTION

◆ ◆ ◆

William Regelson, M.D.

Epidemic diseases of venereal origin are not new to human experience. What is unique about AIDS is that in addition to the thousands infected with the virus, it reminds us constantly of our vulnerability and dramatically alters the sexual or romantic quality of our lives. However, instead of forcing us to confront our ignorance, AIDS, like the bubonic plague that decimated Europe, led many to search for scapegoats instead of enlightenment. Despite this, for the first time, as Arthur Kahn's book documents, those infected in the epidemic disease were able to launch a political fight that gave power to a scientific and social effort to provide relief.

In large measure, the limited gains we have made against AIDS have been the result of anguished individual efforts and community drives organized by those infected by the virus and the people who love them. Heterosexuals owe a debt to the homosexual community. Arthur Kahn's text reviews that struggle and identifies those who took on an unconcerned White House and general public and made the fight against AIDS a national effort.

AIDS bears resemblance to syphilis, our other lethal epidemic venereal disease, which dates back to the fifteenth century. The causative organism was not identified until 1905, followed by a diagnostic test a year later and a therapy developed by Paul Erlich in 1909. Once causative factors or organisms are identified, scientific progress can occur rapidly, and the AIDS-HIV epidemic provides an opportunity to see venereal disease history repeating itself in a modern setting. From the first inkling of an epidemic in 1981, the causative organism was identified rapidly by Montagnier/Gallo in 1983; a diagnostic test followed in 1984; and a much less satisfactory therapeutic approach with azidothymidine in 1987.

In the fifteenth century, it was easier to hold an identifiable group responsible for a disease than to do anything about it. With syphilis, the Spanish and Italians

---

William Regelson is Professor of Medicine, Medical College of Virginia, Virginia Commonwealth University.

blamed the French, and the French blamed the Neapolitans. Today, on the other hand, it is particularly embarrassing to find that the medical struggle against AIDS has been complicated by the prejudices of a political establishment more intent on placing blame than providing for the needs of gays and drug abusers who were the first and chief groups infected with HIV. Only with the spread of AIDS among children and the increasing incidence among adolescents as well as the heterosexual nature of the epidemic in Africa have the press and government focused on the broader implications of this disease.

Despite scientific gains related to the identity and natural history of the disease, despite the appearance of local alternative strategies and attempts to accelerate the foot dragging of the FDA, the scientific effort still needs more effective interdisciplinary approaches. This book speaks to that need. As a cancer researcher, I became involved in the effort in 1985 prompted by earlier work at the Medical College of Virginia related to cancer drugs operating via stimulation of host immunity. In addition, chemotherapy developed against tumor viruses in the early 1970s by the National Cancer Institute (NCI) as part of a multibillion-dollar program coordinated by Timothy E. O'Connor, most recently a director of Biotherapeutics in Franklin, Tennessee, holds clinical promise today against the AIDS virus as potent reverse transcriptase enzyme inhibitors. The data regarding these chemotherapy compounds are probably still sitting on computer tape since the abandonment of the program by the NCI in the late 1970s. One of these compounds, a Merrel (now Marion-Dow) fluorenone derivative, tilorone, is an orally active compound that induces interferon and stimulates immunity. I initiated a limited anticancer clinical trial in the 1970s, but I could not prevail upon people like Sam Broder of the NCI and others in the AIDS establishment to look at these compounds. They had an exaggerated concern for toxicity and ignored the fact that side effects could be controlled along with the additional obvious option to explore a wide range of structural modifications of the parent drug.

Following evidence that the anionic dye suramin and the polyanion dextran sulfate had anti-AIDS virus activity, I unsuccessfully sought to stimulate interest in an investigation of pyran copolymer (Diveema, MVE2), a polyanionic antitumor drug originated at the Medical College of Virginia that had undergone extensive clinical trial as an anticancer immune stimulator (though work with pyran had been conducted by the NCI for many years as a bioresponse modifier). These compounds stimulate interferon, upregulate immunity, inhibit reverse transcriptase and enhance vaccine effectiveness. It is disappointing to find that those who examined suramin as an anti-AIDS drug (an experience described in this book) did not see the relationship between suramin, dextran sulfate and other compounds of this type that had extensive previous clinical trial as immunostimulating, antiviral and anticancer drugs. They merit investigation in AIDS vaccine development.

In 1986 I urged Mathilde Krim and AmFAR (the American Foundation for AIDS Research) to promote a conference to give these neglected alternative AIDS therapies visibility in the scientific community. A small amount of seed money was available from Hercules, the chemical company that held the patent on pyran copolymer, and we were developing plans for a small conference at the Eisenhower Center in Palm Springs. Unfortunately, Mathilde Krim turned the responsibility for organizing this program over to Terry Beirn, an AmFAR general factotum, who would not let us approach the foundation's board of directors. The AIDS struggle includes frustrations by the nongovernmental AIDS establishment as well as by official agencies!

Unfortunately, we have lost four years in the investigation of reverse transcriptase inhibitors because egos were too strong and the competition for funds too severe. Unless those of us not in AIDS research can win over those with reputation and power in the field, old observations of value will have to be rediscovered by younger people entering the field.

In 1984, interested in aging research, I became aware of AL721 and became involved in the promotion of the egg lecithin derivative developed by Meir Shinitzky's group at the Weizmann Institute in Israel. (Its depressing history is presented in detail in this book.) Unfortunately, development rights were given to James Jacobson, a businessman with no scientific background but with an inordinate capacity for creating confusion. AL721 stimulated immune response in aged rodents and in man and had potential activity in stimulating memory function inasmuch as it fluidized cell membranes and revived neural receptors. I served as a consultant to Jacobson in preparing an investigational new drug (IND) geriatrics research program. What made AL721 especially exciting, however, was the fact that it could be considered a food without any need for major FDA involvement. After much procrastination, Jacobson created a company called Ethigen, which under Arnold Lippa, a neuroscientist, offered promise of development. In the middle of a preclinical study evaluating the effects of AL721 on memory in aging rats at the Medical College of Virginia, we were told to return the AL721 to Jacobson as it was not properly constituted. Later we learned that, in fact, Jacobson wanted our supply for a friend in Los Angeles who was dying of AIDS. Such frustrating episodes accompany the history of AL721.

The value of AL721 and related lecithins in memory disorders still needs evaluation as well as appropriate study in immunodeficiency.

Other therapies, neglected though of obvious research potential, include RU 486 or Mifepristone, the French (Roussel-Uclaf) abortifacient, not available for the treatment of AIDS because of pressure from the "right to lifers." It upregulates immunity by blocking corticosteroid action. Nor, strangely, has the value of the spermicide detergent nonoxyenol-9 received adequate attention. While publicizing the value of condoms, AIDS educational efforts ignore nonoxyenol-9, which kills the AIDS virus as well as hepatitis B and other organisms involved in venereal disease. According to the Center for Communicable Diseases, nonoxyenol-9 should be used in conjunction with condoms or with diaphragm vaginal barriers.

Finally, at the Medical College of Virginia we have been developing the steroid hormone dehydroepiandrosterone (DHEA) as an upregulator of immunity. A native hormone produced primarily by the adrenal cortex, DHEA declines with age (80 percent from age 20 to 80); it is practically nonexistent in patients in advanced stages of AIDS. DHEA prevents lethality in mice infected with a coxsackie B enterovirus, herpes type II, encephalitis and a lethal streptococcal infection. It is active by mouth and by subcutaneous injection. It has been tested in Phase I studies in advanced cancer patients and in multiple sclerosis patients and has been shown to improve energy reserves in the chronically ill and to have minimal side effects even at large dosage. Although it may have some direct HIV antiviral activity, its primary action is as an upregulator of immunity. The Elan Corporation of Athlone, Ireland, and Gainesville, Georgia, is testing DHEA in advanced AIDS patients in Amsterdam, San Francisco and New York, but little will be gained except in occasional patients unless DHEA or related steroids are studied in patients in earlier, asymptomatic stages of the disease.

The crucial issue regarding such therapies is presented in persuasive detail in this book. As Arthur Kahn demonstrates, the struggle against AIDS requires a continuous fight against vested interests that have little regard for alternative ideas and against egotists who put self-aggrandizement above a worldwide crisis. We must continue to find ways to catalyze the exploitation of alternative ideas from other disciplines.

Arthur Kahn's book presents the history of the clinical struggle and identifies heroes, many of whom have died fighting for all of us. Their efforts must be recognized. Their struggle is not over.

AIDS,
The
Winter
War

PART I

CHAPTER

"The Mob" Fights Back

I t was only after many setbacks evoking despair and anger during the hectic five years from 1981 (the year of identification of the AIDS disease) to 1986 that the gay community began to shake off its bewilderment and demoralization at the rapid spread of what was at first denominated contemptuously as Gay Related Immune Deficiency (GRID) and only later by the neutral and accurate term Acquired Immune Deficiency Syndrome (AIDS).

During the early 1980s newspapers carried sensationalist headlines about the epidemic. Communities ostentatiously shut down public baths and threatened other gay meeting places. In 1983, contributing to the hysteria, Anthony Fauci, director of the National Institute for Allergies and Infectious Diseases (NIAID), issued an erroneous and irresponsible warning in an editorial in the *Journal of the American Medical Association* entitled "Evidence Suggests Household Contact May Transmit AIDS."

The Moral Majority exulted that sinners were getting their just reward and called for quarantining individuals with the disease. A *Los Angeles Times* poll in December 1985 revealed that 51 percent of Americans were in favor of such a quarantine. Many of those infected with the virus lost their jobs and suffered eviction from their homes as well as abandonment by friends, lovers and family.

In March 1986 William F. Buckley, Jr., editor of the conservative *National Review*, wrote in the *New York Times*: "Everyone detected with AIDS should be tattooed in the upper forearm, to protect common-needle users, and on the buttocks, to prevent the victimization of other homosexuals."

In June 1983 at the United States Conference of Mayors, Margaret Heckler, Secretary of Health and Human Services, announced that AIDS was the department's "number one health priority." Yet five months later, in a report entitled "The Federal Response to AIDS," the House (Weiss) Subcommittee on Intergovernmental Relations and Human Resources charged that the Reagan administration had failed to ensure

3

adequate resources for dealing with its "number one health priority." The Congress had been compelled to override a presidential veto of a supplemental AIDS appropriation of a mere $500,000 for the Centers for Disease Control (CDC); and the National Institutes of Health (NIH) had had to divert funds to AIDS research from projects involving other major diseases.

For fiscal year 1987 the administration proposed cuts on the previous year's appropriations of $14 million for NIH research; $15 million for health care programs; $10 million for antibody testing programs; $2 million for the national AIDS hotline; and $10 million for AIDS education, treatment and related research.

After struggling for six years against official inertia, Mathilde Krim, one of the first scientists to warn of an impending epidemic of enormous proportions, proclaimed: "Everything about this epidemic has been utterly and completely predictable from the very beginning, from the very first day. . . . There are many people who knew exactly what was happening, what would happen and has happened, but no one of importance would listen. They still won't listen. This is an epidemic that could have been contained."

◆ ◆ ◆

Gay activists set about on their own to establish organizations to care for the sick. Thus in its November 1983 report after noting the failure of the Department of Health and Human Resources to disseminate information about AIDS to those at risk for infection and to the national health services community, the House Subcommittee on Intergovernmental Relations and Human Resources praised gay organizations for filling in the void "by establishing hotlines, setting up forums, and developing their own written materials."

In New York City, the major center of the epidemic, the Gay Men's Health Crisis (GMHC) mobilized hundreds of professional and nonprofessional volunteers in manifold educational, social and legal activities and disseminated over 200,000 copies of information booklets. "City officials say they shudder to think of what would have happened in New York," declared the *New York Times* on March 16, 1987, "if the homosexual community had not formed the Gay Men's Health Crisis and other spinoff organizations to care for the sick, educate the healthy and lobby for attention and funds." The article continued with a quote from Dr. Stephen Joseph, the city health commissioner: "When the story of New York's AIDS epidemic is written, that self-help effort will be the bright part of it."

In October 1986 the AIDS community received encouragement from an unexpected ally, Surgeon General C. Everett Koop, whose appointment gay rights organizations had opposed because of his ultraconservative stand on the abortion issue. In his "Report on Acquired Immune Deficiency Syndrome," Koop declared:

> At the beginning of the AIDS epidemic many Americans had little sympathy for
> people with AIDS. The feeling was that somehow people from certain groups

"deserved" their illness. Let us put such feelings behind us. We are fighting a disease, not people. . . . The country must face this epidemic as a unified society. We must prevent the spread of AIDS while at the same time preserving our humanity and intimacy.

Koop went on to warn of a devastating impact from the epidemic: "By the end of 1991 an estimated 145,000 patients with AIDS will need health and supportive services at a total cost of between $8 and $16 billion. . . . With proper information and education, as many as 12,000 to 14,000 could be saved in 1991 from death."

The Lavender Hill Mob

A dramatic manifestation of reviving militancy in the gay community during the mid-eighties, the Lavender Hill Mob captured national attention and not only shook up the establishment but also provided a powerful impetus to aggressive action by members of the gay community and their allies. The Mob was an informal group of a dozen or so radical gay activists, four of whom were women. Providing the vision for the group was Brooklyn-born Marty Robinson, 44, a typical sixties activist, an authentic hippie as a youth (and still a hippie twenty years later). He had dropped out of Brooklyn College because he did not believe that he could find in books what he wanted to learn.

Participating in the 1969 melee at the Stonewall gay bar in Greenwich Village when infuriated gays battled police raiders, Marty said to himself, "This I understand, this is self-respect." Subsequently Marty helped organize gay activist groups, which, he says, "developed the 'zap' [a dramatic, attention-getting action] to an art and put gay people out in public view."

Only after Stonewall did Bill Bahlman, a few years younger than Marty, begin to think, "I have to pay my dues." He became chairman of the Gay Movement Committee of the Gay Activist Alliance, and as a member also of its speakers' bureau he addressed student groups throughout the city. By 1974 he experienced temporary burnout in his gay activism. Becoming involved again late in 1985, he discovered that the leadership of gay organizations was fearful of mass demonstrations. He was ready for the Mob.

Raised in conservative Pennsylvania Dutch country, Henry Yaeger, at 56 the oldest of the "mobsters," participated in a St. John's University faculty strike in support of members of the Philosophy Department dismissed for failing to promote the institution's prescribed Catholic line. He decided he was ready for gay activism when at a GLAAD (Gay and Lesbian Action Against Discrimination) demonstration in December 1985, Marty Robinson, dramatically brash, arrived with a tractor trailer instead of the four-foot-by-eight-foot platform authorized by the police.

Though not loath to claim credit for actions organized by "radicals" that obtained coverage in the news media, leaders of the Gay and Lesbian Alliance and of the Coalition for Gay and Lesbian Rights were wary of aggressive demonstrations and were discomfited when on July 1, 1986, the "radicals" persuaded 3,000 people at a Sheridan Square rally protesting a Supreme Court ruling on sodomy to block traffic. Three days later, on July 4, Marty and his friends led a march of 7,000 people from Battery Park at the southern tip of Manhattan up to Greenwich Village, and on August 11 they assembled 2,500 gays to demonstrate at Lincoln Center. "The gay community was ready for direct confrontation," says Marty. "We merely provided the leadership."

In the fall of 1986 having decided they could function more effectively as an independent entity, the activists sought a name appropriate to their particular activism. "Lavender" defined them as gays. "Mob" characterized them as aggressive activists. *The Lavender Hill Mob*, the title of a well-known British comic film, conveyed the imagination and humor of the zap.

The Mob's first zap occurred on October 16, 1986 at the annual Alfred E. Smith dinner, the leading social event of the Roman Catholic New York establishment, attended by John Cardinal O'Connor, the governor, the mayor and other celebrities. Marty Robinson had sent a check for $3,200 for eight reservations. (He stopped payment on the check after the event!) As U.S. Ambassador to the United Nations Vernon Walters began to orate about the "evil empire," the Lavender Hill Mob jumped up in a body and cried out, "Gays and Lesbians will not be silenced." Quickly they distributed leaflets. The press conference they had announced in advance did not take place, but the event did break into the press.

On Sunday, November 2, the Mob conducted a zap at St. Patrick's Cathedral in protest of a Vatican encyclical condemning homosexuality. While forty-five people stood outside, including two Mobsters dressed as priests prepared to read statements by various Catholic dignitaries, nine others inside the cathedral stood up and unfurled the Lavender Hill Mob banner as soon as Cardinal O'Connor began his sermon. After a few minutes, they marched out in silence. Their action was announced on breaks during television broadcasts of football games.

On November 20, in one of their first zaps specifically on the AIDS issue, ten Mobsters occupied the New York offices of Senator Alphonse D'Amato and plastered mock arrest warrants over the walls charging the senator with 15,345 deaths for not speaking out on the AIDS pandemic.

On February 24, 1987, exhausting their savings for airfare and accommodations, the Mob flew to Atlanta to zap a two-day CDC conference promoting the Reagan administration's policy of mandatory AIDS testing. At the opening plenary session, the Mobsters took places throughout the hall for a swift distribution of bright yellow leaflets with the slogan "Test Drugs, Not People." In a symbolic indictment of the administration for failing to mount an organized campaign against the epidemic, Eric Perez and Michael Petrelis appeared in concentration camp uniforms adorned with the pink triangle, the Nazi symbol for gays. Throughout the conference, cameras flashed and reporters crowded about for interviews. During open microphone sessions, the Mobsters were always in line.

At the final session, when Walter Dowdle, deputy director of the CDC, was delivering closing remarks, the group unfurled the Lavender Hill Mob banner adorned with a slogan about genocide. "Here you're talking about testing [for the AIDS virus]," shouted the Mobsters, "and what about testing other drugs? What about Ribavirin, what about AL721?"

The zap was reported throughout the United States as well as in numerous other countries. Bill Bahlman appeared on the CNN national cable program "Crossfire," and each of the five Mobsters enjoyed an average of fifteen to twenty interviews with the press per day. Within weeks of the Atlanta conference zaps, a group of graphic artists in New York put up posters throughout the city with the slogan "Silence Equals Death" under a pink triangle.

In March, too, Larry Kramer in the *New York Native* attacked establishment gay organizations for timidity in confronting government lethargy. A former executive at Columbia Pictures and United Artists and an Academy Award winner as writer and producer of the film version of D. H. Lawrence's *Women in Love*, Kramer was also the author of *The Normal Heart*, a successful play about AIDS. Kramer enjoyed widespread prestige in the gay community, and when he delivered an impassioned appeal at the New York Gay and Lesbian Community Center for a revival of the militancy of the post-Stonewall era, he inspired the audience then and there to organize a new mass activist organization, ACT UP (AIDS Coalition to Unleash Power).

With the collaboration of the Lavender Hill Mob, over the next months in rapid succession ACT UP conducted demonstrations on Wall Street and at the Federal Plaza against procrastination by the Food and Drug Administration in authorizing new therapies; at the main post office on the April 15 income tax deadline, demanding additional federal appropriations for AIDS research; and at the offices of Northeast Orient Airlines for refusing to transport PWAs.

ACT UP was to become the leading AIDS activist organization, with chapters throughout the country. In April 1988, at a hearing of the Weiss House subcommittee, Iris Long, testifying as an ACT UP spokesperson, defined ACT UP's goals as follows: "to bring the medical and political issues surrounding AIDS before the public and government officials for dialogue and resolution, to focus media attention on the government's mismanagement of the AIDS crisis, the unavailability of promising treatments, the exorbitant price of drugs, the lack of prophylaxis treatment for opportunistic infections, the underenrollment in government clinical trials and the lack of an up-to-date registry of trials."

◆ ◆ ◆

By June 1987, when 6,000 people from many nations assembled in Washington for the third annual International Conference on AIDS, the Mob was well known to government officials and to the media. At the opening session three Mobsters appeared dressed in white laboratory coats adorned with lavender crosses. On their shirts under pink triangles they displayed the new activist motto, "Silence Equals Death."

With hundreds of gay activists mobilized by the newly organized ACT UP demonstrating noisily outside the hall, the press and government officials anticipated some outrageous zap by the Mobsters within. After distributing leaflets with the heading "Reagan Administration Fears Human Sexuality More Than AIDS," however, the Mobsters quietly took seats in the second row, in clear view of the podium. Mobster Bill Bahlman found himself directly in front of Anthony Fauci. Director of NIAID and head of NIH's AIDS research program, Fauci had been hailed by Ted Koppel on ABC's "Nightline" as "America's leading expert on AIDS." Bill asked Fauci whether the Mob would be upset by what Vice President George Bush, the keynote speaker, was about to say. "You'll probably like his remarks," said Fauci, "if he sticks to what I wrote for him." In fact, Bush reiterated the call for mandatory testing, a call for which President Reagan had been booed the previous evening at a dinner of the American Foundation for AIDS Research. Hundreds of public health officials now joined the Mob in booing the vice president.

Unaware that his microphone was still live, Bush muttered, "What is that? Some gay group out there?" His remark, heard by the entire assemblage, provided newspaper headlines.

Later that day, when the Mobsters resisted the efforts of security police to stop them from distributing leaflets, Dr. James B. Wyngaarden, director of NIH and the chairman of the conference, pleaded, "Now, guys!" Marty Robinson responded, "Now, Wyngaarden! Don't get in our way! We're distributing information." "Okay, guys," replied Wyngaarden, "but, please, don't bust up the conference."

Besieged by reporters and registrants, the Mob distributed a total of 15,000 leaflets, a different one each day. One was headlined: "Are You Now or Have You Ever Been Sero-positive?" The Mob received so many requests for buttons with the slogan "Silence Equals Death" that they sent to New York for an additional 800. An official of the Hawaii Department of Health reached into his pocket and handed Marty a $20 bill as "a contribution to the extraordinary work you're doing."

On the day of the final session a Mob leaflet called upon the registrants to "Stand for Medicine and Science."

With a hyperbolical eulogy of Secretary of Health and Human Services Otis Bowen, the final speaker of the conference, as a politician, a football hero and a devoted public servant, Assistant Secretary Robert E. Windom sought desperately to soften the impact of the zap everyone was anticipating. The longer he spoke and the more hyperbolical his praise, the more the audience chuckled. When Bowen rose to speak, three Mobsters stood up, turned and faced the audience. Hundreds of registrants rose with them, many booing and jeering. Marty looked at Food and Drug Administration Commissioner Frank Young and saw his face drop.

All the television networks carried the zap, as did newspapers in many countries.

This bold and dramatic action symbolized the new resolution and militancy within the gay community, roused in a life-and-death struggle against the AIDS epidemic.

Marty Robinson died of AIDS on March 19, 1992.

CHAPTER 2

Two Therapies, Two FDA–NIH Approaches

AZT: The Official Therapy

> In 1984 . . . people were dying without intervention. . . . We knew that if we could find a drug already in the market-place we could get something very quickly and with little cost. We had to find a company that would find it in its interest to develop an AIDS drug. . . . We needed companies to see that there was money to be made here.

Thus in 1987 Samuel Broder, director of the National Cancer Institute clinical oncology program, recalled how in reaction to intensifying congressional and public criticism of bureaucratic inertia, NIH began to encourage pharmaceutical companies to undertake AIDS research.

Broder found a company, Burroughs Wellcome, a mammoth multinational corporation able to gamble tens of millions on a project in which "there was money to be made." A firm with a long and close association with NIH and FDA and broad contacts in medical and hospital circles, Burroughs Wellcome commanded a large, specialized staff and almost unlimited resources as well as a plant with its own laboratories, production facilities and publicity services.

According to a comprehensive story in the *Washington Post* of September 15, 1987 by reporter Mark H. Furstenberg, Burroughs Wellcome researchers scanned the half-million experimental drugs catalogued in FDA computers and selected several hundred compounds as the most likely candidates for in vitro testing by the NIH. In February 1985 one of the Burroughs' submissions showed promise—AZT. Developed in 1964 with government funding by a scientist at the Michigan Cancer Foundation, AZT had been discarded as ineffective as a cancer therapy and had not been patented. Doses administered to AIDS patients hospitalized at the NIH brought results that were, according to FDA and NIH officials, "astonishing."

Instead of undertaking a conservative double-blind study with patients in earlier stages of the disease, in February 1986 Burroughs Wellcome in coordination with NCI began testing AZT right off with very sick patients, a bold gamble that Lowell T. Harmison, deputy secretary of Health and Human Services, hailed as an example of "the way the capitalist system is supposed to work." By September, two months after the last patient was enrolled in the study, 13 of 281 people had died, while the others were improving markedly. It was discovered that all those who had died, with one exception, had been on a placebo. Adjudging these results conclusive, NIH officials ended the test and presented the drug to FDA for approval.

In April 1987, admitting that AZT was not a cure but insisting that it extended the life of people with AIDS, FDA Commissioner Frank Young boasted to a House subcommittee of the fastest approval of an ethical pharmaceutical in FDA history: "Instead of taking its average [review time of] 760 to 790 days, [FDA] took 108 days."

Privately Burroughs Wellcome expressed its gratitude to Dr. Broder for his collaboration. On May 23, 1985 Kathy L. Russell, the administrative officer at Dr. Broder's Clinical Oncology Program at the National Cancer Institute, wrote Dr. Sandra N. Lehrman of Burroughs Wellcome:

> As per our telephone conversation, the National Cancer Institute would be
> happy to receive a donation from Burroughs Wellcome in support of
> Dr. Broder's work. The check should be made payable to the National Cancer
> Institute and the letter accompanying the donation to my attention should
> indicate that this is a gift to the National Cancer Institute in support of
> Dr. Broder's efforts and should be used to provide fellow support to Dr. Broder's
> laboratory.

The company promptly sent a check for $55,000 "'in support of Dr. Samuel Broder's Laboratory's work on AIDS." On July 11, 1985, however, Russell returned the check. Because of new regulations, she declared, the NCI could not "administer fellow support with donations made directly to the Institute." She asked the company to make out a new check payable to the Foundation for the Advancement of Education in the Sciences, "a non-profit, non-federal organization which administers private grants and donations to fellows and students interested in scientific research." The company sent a second check, made out as Russell instructed.

On October 1, 1987 charging that the correspondence between Kathy Russell and Burroughs Wellcome, disclosed under a Freedom of Information request, exposed how "Broder encouraged Burroughs Wellcome to 'donate' money to support Dr. Broder's work," Leonard Graff, legal director of the National Gay Rights Advocates, noted that the "encouragement of the 'donation' occurred at the same time as the corporation gained the designation of AZT as an orphan drug," a designation that grants the manufacturer of a drug with a limited clientele exclusive authority to market that drug for a period of five years.

While privately rewarding Broder for his assistance, publicly Burroughs Wellcome denied any NIH contribution to the development of AZT. On January 14, 1987, disturbed by a Burroughs Wellcome release to the Associated Press, Broder sent a letter to David Barry, the corporation's vice president for research, in which he objected to an "implication that the development of AZT was somehow unintentional." The development of AZT, Broder insisted, "took place because of a very intentional collaboration between the company and the National Cancer Institute."

Broder also took exception to the contention that it was the company that "had the drug tested on human viruses." "All of us," Broder commented, "are very happy and proud that we were able to generate data demonstrating the activity of AZT against an array of pathogenic human retroviruses. . . . Providing the necessary technology required intellectual and, at the time, possible physical risks on the part of the NCI scientists working with HTLV-III [the AIDS virus, dangerous to handle in laboratory procedures]. These facts do not seem to be encompassed by the expression 'had the drug tested' in the context of the article."

Two months later on March 19, 1987 in a further angry letter, Broder expressed chagrin at the testimony of a Burroughs Wellcome vice president before a congressional committee "that AZT was developed within the company with little substantive contribution by others." On the contrary, declared Broder:

> The development of AZT would not have occurred without the substantial commitment (and transfer) of government technology. . . . Indeed, your position ignores the entire [NCI] Viral Cancer Program. . . . [t]he specific development of AZT as a medicinal anti-retroviral agent required a substantial commitment of resources and personnel, not to say the assumptions of certain risks on the part of government scientists.

Broder did not mention that NCI even made available gratis government stocks of thymidine, an expensive substance that was an essential ingredient of AZT.

On April 12, 1987 the *New York Times* quoted Anthony Fauci of NIAID as complaining "that Burroughs Wellcome literally ha[d] complete control of what [did] or [did] not get done in trials involving AZT . . . sponsored by the National Institutes of Health."

When Lowell T. Harmison, deputy secretary of Health and Human Services, applied for a patent for AZT on behalf of the Department of Health and Human Services, he discovered that Burroughs Wellcome, apparently more sophisticated than he as to "the way that capitalism is supposed to work," had jumped the gun and secured the patent for itself.

Licensed by the government to manufacture and distribute the drug, Burroughs Wellcome had a free hand in setting the maximum price the market could bear— a price that ranged as high as $13,000 for a year's supply, the highest price ever charged for a pharmaceutical drug. When at congressional hearings in July 1987 Representative Ron Wyden of Oregon snapped, "Why didn't you set the price at $100,000 per patient?" corporation president T. E. Haigler, Jr., ignoring the congressman's sarcasm, replied: "We are trying to set the price based on what we think is a reasonable price for this drug that is shown to be effective for this particular disease."

By September 1987 some 10,000 AIDS patients were taking AZT on prescription, and another 2,000 were obtaining it through participation in clinical trials. The *Wall Street Journal* of September 11, 1987 quoted a securities analyst as estimating a 60 percent profit margin for Burroughs, adding: "With an envisioned doubling of AZT's user pool, there is a lot of money to be made."

In 1986 and 1987 Burroughs Wellcome, it is fair to note, did provide a supply of AZT to a limited number of patients, perhaps fifty, on a compassionate plea basis.

AZT: Some Unanswered Questions

Although encouraged by the rapid approval of AZT and hopeful that this expeditious procedure would be applied to other promising AIDS therapies, the AIDS community was disturbed by certain aspects of the testing procedures and suspicious about the collaboration between NIH and FDA and Burroughs Wellcome.

The public had not been informed that the FDA review panel that approved AZT was not unanimous in its decision. Michael Lange, a consultant to the panel, expressed opposition to the approval, and Itzak Brook, chairman of the panel, was outvoted by his colleagues on the decision to recommend rapid authorization of the compound. Other experts, too, began to voice their doubts.

In a letter in the September 1987 issue of the *New England Journal of Medicine*, Dr. Seymour Cohen, a preeminent biochemist of Woods Hole, Massachusetts, posed questions in regard to the toxicity of AZT, noting that no information had been supplied about possible damage to normal cells and possible carcinogenic effects of the drug.

Because of such expressions of concern about the drug, ACT UP in New York and Project Inform in San Francisco asked Dr. Joseph Sonnabend, a well-known New York AIDS physician and a scientist of distinction, to analyze both FDA reports on the AZT test data (obtained by Project Inform under the Freedom of Information Act) and additional data published in the July 23, 1987 issue of the *New England Journal of Medicine*.

Dr. Sonnabend questioned whether the clinical data on AZT accumulated over a mere sixteen-week period demonstrated that AZT by virtue of its anti-retroviral action was responsible for the results claimed. Of the 144 patients receiving AZT and the 137 on placebo in the multicenter controlled trial, he noted, only fifteen completed twenty-four weeks of trial and twenty-seven completed twenty-three weeks. Enrolment proceeded from February through June of 1986. The placebo was discontinued in September when it was found that nineteen (not thirteen, as originally announced) on placebo died compared with only one on AZT.

Furthermore, according to Sonnabend, the causes of death had not been properly documented. "On the case report forms for the patients who died," FDA reviewers admitted, "there are only a few which report biopsy or culture proof of the clinical diagnosis reported. No actual histology, pathology or culture reports are attached." "It is therefore impossible," Sonnabend commented, "to ascertain if any of the above reported deaths might have been preventable, at least within the duration of the study, by means less toxic than AZT."

In addition, patients enrolled in the controlled study were restricted to AZT or the placebo and deprived, for example, of prophylaxis against pneumocystis carinii pneumonia (PCP), the most common cause of death among those infected with HIV. Eight died of PCP, according to the *New England Journal of Medicine*; four, according to the FDA review. No information was provided in the case reports regarding the treatment accorded the patients who died.

FDA reviewers admitted that "the treatment groups unblinded themselves early" and that this unblinding "could have resulted in bias in the work up of patients."

Since all the placebo subjects were offered AZT in September 1986 the double-blind study was discontinued before it measured the duration of the effect of the treatment on survival. On the basis of the report of seven deaths by December and eleven more deaths by February 1987 over and above the nineteen during the double-blind study, Sonnabend concluded that "in view of its toxicity and particularly the possibility of cumulative toxicity, the administration of AZT beyond 16 weeks may not be justified with the information currently available."

Reviewers appointed by FDA also admitted that "the bias toward reporting [adverse drug experiences] as [disease or drug related] . . . was altered during the course of the study from a 'bias' towards 'overreporting' them as possible adverse drug events at the beginning of the study, to 'overreporting' them as presumptively disease-associated events later in the study. . . . Adverse experiences were sometimes crossed out months after initially recorded." They concluded, "This type of action typifies the confusion concerning the appropriate way to record symptoms and possible adverse reactions and casts some doubt on the validity of the analyses of these parameters."

Testifying in February 1988 at hearings of the Presidential Commission, Dr. Barry Gingell, director of the Medical Information Program of the Gay Men's Health Crisis, noted the expense of AZT both financially and in terms of toxicity. He cited a study of the original AZT recipients a year later as providing sobering figures: "Fully 40% of patients experience serious hematologic toxicity after one year, and 25% have to discontinue use entirely. The magic drug Retrovir [AZT]," he went on to charge, ". . . foisted on the public as a triumph against AIDS is actually turning out to be a cumulative poison . . . creat[ing] its own set of serious hematologic problems, which may in fact contribute to the disease rather than moderate it. . . . AZT causes serious bone marrow suppression, resulting in lowered red and white cells in the blood. . . . AZT-induced neutropenia may be a contributing factor for the increasing numbers of bacterial infections now being seen in AIDS. . . . AZT has no effect on blocking cell-to-cell HIV infection." Dr. Gingell concluded with the admonition that "because of these serious shortcomings, AZT should actually be considered only as a prototype antiviral drug."

With AZT still the single drug authorized by FDA for AIDS therapy and with disquieting questions emerging about it, the general AIDS community was made aware that more than zaps were required to prod government agencies to quicker and more effective action against the epidemic. It was clear that to meet FDA and NIH on their own ground the AIDS community would have to develop a sophistication about the therapies and about their testing and approval and involve itself in legal actions as well as protest demonstrations to compel government agencies and pharmaceutical companies to expedite the discovery, approval and distribution of new therapies at costs that patients and public health agencies could bear.

The Ribavirin Affair

The AIDS community complained that in "putting all its eggs in one basket [AZT]," NIH was failing to investigate or was investigating with reluctance other promising unauthorized therapies in wide use among individuals infected with HIV.

Unlike AZT, relegated during two decades to a computer listing as a failed therapy for cancer, Ribavirin had a twelve-year active history of success as a therapy with a number of different human viral diseases and was licensed for medical use in over thirty countries. In addition, according to a 1986 publication of the American Foundation for AIDS Research, side effects of Ribavirin had been found to be treatable and reversible.

After in vitro studies at the Centers for Disease Control in 1984 demonstrated that Ribavirin inhibited replication of HIV, PWAs, especially on the West Coast, began to cross the Mexican border in rapidly swelling numbers to obtain supplies of the unauthorized therapy.

Martin Delaney's lover was one of those who crossed the border to buy Ribavirin. Within weeks he noticed a remarkable change in his condition. His subsequent therapeutic experience helped prepare Martin to become one of the leading spokesmen for the AIDS community.

In 1978, at the age of 34, Martin moved to San Francisco, where he worked as a consultant to *Fortune* 500 companies in the development of educational materials and corporate publications. With PWAs like his lover buying "underground" drugs, often at great cost, or concocting them in their own kitchens, Martin, like other gay activists, began to suspect that the federal bureaucracy was withholding or failing to test substances that seemed to be helping a lot of people.

In 1984 in the laundry room in Martin's house, Martin and Joe Brewer, a San Francisco psychotherapist with a number of HIV patients, set up a work table with a computer and filing cabinets, and under the organization name Project Inform they began to provide advice on unauthorized treatments they investigated.

Early in 1985 a San Francisco organization, Mobilization Against AIDS, invited

Martin to debate a representative of FDA on the issue of across-the-border purchase of AIDS treatments. To Martin's astonishment, the FDA spokesman was not only unfamiliar with any of the drugs that Martin mentioned but was, in fact, unaware of the widespread dissemination of unauthorized drugs.

Upon being invited to a clinic for Kaposi's sarcoma (an opportunistic disease associated with HIV infection) at the University of California at San Francisco, Martin and his colleague described their Project Inform activities to seventy of the top researchers in the city. The warm reception indicated the possibility of useful collaboration between AIDS activists and scientists and physicians. Complaining of a lack of research money and of bureaucratic NIH controls, the seventy researchers offered suggestions, advice and encouragement.

Martin and Joe won agreement from ICN (also called Viratek), the manufacturer of Ribavirin, for an adjustment in price for group purchases in Mexico and for the allocation of a portion of the company's profits to research. Upon receiving a substantial subsidy from ICN, Martin and Joe opened an office, installed a telephone and initiated a survey of some 120 individuals who had been taking Ribavirin. The results of the survey were positive.

In December 1985 FDA approved a Phase II multicenter clinical trial to assess the efficacy of Ribavirin at two early stages of HIV infection—lymphadenopathy (LAS) and AIDS Related Complex (ARC). Upon completion of the LAS tests in December 1986 Dr. Richard J. Whitley, professor of pediatrics and microbiology at the University of Alabama at Birmingham and chairman of a Data Safety Monitoring Board Committee composed of independent authorities, reported that the committee adjudged these studies "to be among the most complex, long running, double-blind, placebo-controlled trials in the history of infectious diseases." The committee recommended a continuation of the trials.

Three months after receiving the test results, FDA on April 10 rejected an ICN request for a treatment IND—a designation of Ribavirin as an "investigational new drug"—which would have permitted broader-based testing of Ribavirin with LAS patients as well as administration of the drug on a compassionate basis to life-threatened AIDS patients. Three days later, challenging the randomization in the selection of patients in the 1986 tests and raising questions as to the safety of the drug, FDA placed Ribavirin on "clinical hold." On April 29, testifying before the Weiss congressional subcommittee, Commissioner Young declared that he and his colleagues had "really had no difficulty [in rejecting] a request for a treatment IND for Ribavirin." In addition to questioning the safety of the drug, he declared, "we were also concerned that clearly it provided no therapeutic benefit." (In fact, in the LAS multicenter clinical trial of 163 patients, ten people in the group taking a placebo progressed to AIDS, whereas none receiving the drug did so.) Young hinted at financial interests in ICN among some of the researchers and ordered an investigation of the research centers involved in the study.

When Martin Delaney telephoned the scientists involved in the trials, he found them in a fury. They recalled the eagerness with which FDA had accepted data of AZT clinical tests in which several of their number had participated. All denied any financial connection with ICN. Peter Mansell, director of the AIDS hospital in Houston, Peter Hazeltine at the University of California at Los Angeles and Richard Roberts at Cornell were unanimous in their conviction of the integrity of the trials. They insisted that the efficacy of Ribavirin had been clearly demonstrated and were angry not only at FDA's rejection of their findings but at aspersions on their competence and ethics.

ICN then assembled an independent board, including preeminent scientists, to review the FDA ruling. After studying the FDA statistical analysis as well as an analysis of the FDA report by Dr. Alan Forsythe, statistician for ICN, the board members expressed unanimity in "finding no basis in fact" for any of the criticisms by FDA. One of the scientists rejected FDA evaluator Dr. Ellen Cooper's "suggestion that patients with Kaposi's sarcoma should be analyzed differently from other patients"; another of the independent evaluators insisted "there is some prima facie evidence of some benefit" from the drug and decried the "FDA's seemingly rather mechanical attitude"; still another scoffed that "most of [the FDA reviewer's] suggestions are in the direction of reducing the chance of showing significance irrespective of the study of data at hand."

On June 30, 1987 Dr. Earl Shelp, professor of medical ethics at the Center for Ethics, Medicine and Public Issues at the College of Medicine of Baylor University and a member of the Data Safety Monitoring Board that reviewed the Ribavirin clinical study, wrote to Dr. Robert E. Windom, assistant secretary for health, that he found no justification for FDA's withholding of approval of Ribavirin. He warned that "statistical hair-splitting should have no place where literally millions of lives hang in the balance." Similarly, after an investigation at the University of Southern California Medical Center, one of the institutions participating in the Ribavirin study, an FDA field representative declared, "I did not find any bias in that regard in the study at all. I found the randomization was acceptable."

On June 1, 1987 Eppler, Guerin and Turner, a Wall Street investment firm, issued a sharply worded report of its investigation of the dispute. "The NIH obviously is interested," the report declared, "in getting its own product [AZT] on the market ahead of Ribavirin in order to justify its taxpayer-based funding and to ensure the success of its own products." The report found it ironic that the FDA commissioner should show such concern with Ribavirin's possible toxicity after approving AZT, the toxicity of which it described as "almost worse than AIDS."

To the FDA's undocumented accusations of possible stock manipulation, the Wall Street investigators offered a blunt denunciation of FDA's leaks to "certain stock market players" regarding concerns for the safety and efficacy of Ribavirin as a "blatant attempt to drive down the price of ICN stock." The leak of confidential information from within FDA, the report continued, "evidences an apparent disdain for the proper and fair review to which new drugs should be entitled. Such disdain is particularly damaging in the extremely sensitive environment surrounding AIDS research, where even a whisper of hope or despair reverberates throughout a stricken community."

The report further noted the irony in FDA's placing a hold on further Ribavirin trials while simultaneously working out an understanding with the Customs Office to allow U.S. citizens to import Ribavirin from Mexico. Under this "cynical" arrangement private citizens were permitted "to perform unsupervised 'do it yourself' experiments with unknown dosages of Ribavirin." On the other hand, FDA refused to grant a treatment IND for Ribavirin, "which would at least allow further testing of Ribavirin under scrupulously supervised conditions."

Upon receiving a letter from Martin Delaney questioning aspects of the controversy, Commissioner Young invited him to Washington, and on July 28, 1987, Martin gained further insight into the workings of the government bureaucracy. Scheduled to last forty-five minutes, the meeting between Martin and ten of Young's FDA and NIH associates continued for three hours. To Delaney, FDA and NIH officials appeared far less categorical in their rejection of Ribavirin than they had been during the previous six months. They blamed the president of the company for problems leading to the current dispute. (Delaney knew the head of the firm to be an aggressive and cantankerous individual, clumsy and difficult in negotiations.)

When suspicions of stock manipulations in the company's history were posed during the discussion, Martin suggested that such a charge was a matter for the Securities and Exchange Commission, not for FDA. If Ribavirin was useful, Martin insisted, everybody lost if testing and promotion were not handled properly. "You accuse the ICN people of running around and promoting their products," he declared. "To us Sam Broder seems to have been promoting the hell out of AZT before anyone tested it." At the mention of Broder's name, the group burst into laughter. (Clearly, there were strains within officialdom!)

Martin was told that FDA decisions were ultimately made by the two reviewers present at the meeting, Drs. Ellen Cooper and Nazim Moledina. "Both look as though they had just finished college," Martin reported. "They were not the seasoned experts I had hoped to find when I went to Washington."

When Martin asked where these inexperienced reviewers obtained information for their evaluations and whom they consulted regarding their rulings, he was told that they spent their time at NIAID and took cues from director Anthony S. Fauci and his associates.

"We've got the fox investigating the chickens," commented Martin.

Three months after this meeting, on October 10, 1987, admitting that no safety problem existed and retracting the earlier charge of errors in randomization in the clinical tests of 1986 but offering no apology for the defamatory accusations leveled against researchers, Young lifted the six-month hold on Ribavirin. Trials were immediately initiated at Cornell University Medical Center and by the U.S. Army, which investigated Ribavirin as a low-toxicity alternative to AZT.

"FDA Commissioner Young," commented *Project Inform Perspectives*, the organ of the office established some years earlier by Martin and his colleague, "should be fired for his handling of Ribavirin matters."

Ellen Cooper, the FDA reviewer who bore much of the responsibility for frustrating the progress of Ribavirin in the FDA authorization process, was not fired for her apparently hasty evaluation of the drug. She was promoted head of AIDS Drug Evaluation.

During his meeting with Frank Young and Young's associates, Martin Delaney asked, "What are you doing to help a Ribavirin or an AL721 [another AIDS therapy in wide use, discussed in forthcoming chapters] get developed?"

"We just work on the drugs that we think are the most promising, and private industry can do what it wants" was the reply.

"Is it up to me then," demanded Martin, "to come here to intercede for the development of drugs that people need?"

Martin's challenge was met with silence, but he was more aware of how to focus his future activity in the AIDS struggle.

Pending further FDA action, PWAs continued to purchase Ribavirin in Mexico, and FDA continued to permit its importation. But by the spring of 1988 the price had increased more than 3,000 percent. When Barry Gingell, director of medical information for GMHC, was asked why, having been forced to abandon treatment with AZT because of its severe side effects, he did not renew treatment with Ribavirin, which had proved effective with him, he replied: "I'm too exhausted to make the trip to Mexico, and the price is now out of my reach."

Within the general AIDS struggle, the efficacy of Ribavirin as a therapeutic agent against HIV infection (still undetermined in 1992) may have been less significant than whether FDA and NIH bureaucracy were applying different standards in approving AZT from those they applied with other drugs. Was there collusion between government agencies and Burroughs Wellcome in preventing an equally rapid testing and authorization of other therapies?

As for FDA's charge of stock manipulation with Ribavirin (a charge never pressed in the courts or through the Securities and Exchange Commission), stock manipulation with drugs is not an unfamiliar phenomenon in the U.S. pharmaceutical industry. The May 8, 1988 "Durant and Livermore Cutten and Bliss Report," an investment newsletter, thus described the stock manipulation of a certain Greenwich Pharmaceuticals:

> Since at least 1974 it has been in the drug development business, relying since 1976 on a patented compound it trademarked as Therafectin to raise money. And raise money it has—something on the order of $28,000,000. . . . No product sales so far because it is still, 12 years later, trying to get its act together

and submit the drug to the FDA for approval to sell as a Rheumatoid Arthritis palliative.

> . . . a drug guru . . . explained [that] all of the patents describe essentially the same compound, which consists of two proven anti-virals already on the market. . . . Instead of patenting a new substance that could be easily copied, [the company has] found a way to patent proven antivirals that are already being marketed.

> . . . Looking at the record of money raised and stock sold by insiders, a suspicious person might believe that selling paper rather than drugs was the main concern of the promoters. Having a drug that permits periodic releases of good test results . . . and a *patent* provides a fool proof way to tell the truth to snake oil investors and still get their money. Very, very clever.

It may never be known how much AIDS research was stymied by similar examples of corporate profiteering. The story of AL721, for two years a popular AIDS therapy among PWAs, however, offers insights into pharmaceutical maneuvering.

CHAPTER 3

PWAs Undertake AIDS Research

The Consumer Treatment Initiative

As early as 1983 dramatist and gay activist Larry Kramer was urging CDC to collaborate with the gay community in AIDS research and epidemiology. "We have volunteers at the Gay Men's Health Crisis," he said; "we can do the intake and the interviewing, we can provide the statistics." His suggestion ignored, Kramer complained that "all these people think that they alone have knowledge. They know nothing about our community, yet they call the shots in controlling our lives."

Unwilling to be stymied by lack of interest at CDC in a collaboration with the AIDS community, in the fall of 1986 the New York Persons with AIDS Coalition instructed two PWAs, Ron Najman and Michael Callen, to invite Drs. Mathilde Krim and Joseph Sonnabend to join in drafting a proposal for a "Consumer Treatment Initiative." Even before the definition of the disease in 1981 Krim and Sonnabend had been leaders in the AIDS struggle. Mathilde Krim had studied at the Weizmann Institute in Israel and earned a reputation for her research with interferon, a new drug with manifold medical possibilities. From television programs and public meetings on AIDS Krim had become well-known throughout the nation and internationally as a spokesman for the AIDS community. With quiet dignity, she exposed misconceptions about the virus and campaigned to educate the government and the public as to the peril of the epidemic and as to ways of preventing its spread.

Upon coming to the United States from his native South Africa, Sonnabend served as a professor and researcher at the Albert Einstein College of Medicine, at Mt. Sinai Medical School, at New York's Downstate Medical School and finally at the Uniformed Services University of Health Sciences in Bethesda, Maryland. He became disillusioned in his teaching experience. "American students don't understand that learning is hard work," he declared; "it's not fun." Discussions in staff meetings, he discovered, revolved about grants rather than what he considered to be basic professional matters. In 1979, abandoning his teaching career, Sonnabend underwent a major change in his life. "If a month earlier," he declared, "I had been told that I would be in private practice, I would have found the idea ludicrous."

For Sonnabend AIDS did not "occur out of the blue." When the epidemic was defined in 1981, he associated it with his experiences with patients suffering from lymph node enlargements and from repeated multiple infections. He set the development of the new disease within the social environment of sexual freedom and experimentation of the sixties and seventies. AIDS, he concluded, was not caused by a single agent; it developed out of a variety of factors impacting on the immune system. It was the result of a process that prepared the way for the virus. He published several papers expressing his views—papers that, because of their unorthodoxy, earned him more abuse than respect.

Badgered by neighbors alarmed at the stream of AIDS patients coming to his door, an experience that received broad coverage in the New York press, Sonnabend was forced to move his office. He found space in a tenement building.

Already in the early eighties Sonnabend had 4,000 cases in his files. By 1987 he had suffered at least a hundred deaths among his patients.

According to a proposal issued on November 11, 1986 by the two PWAs and Drs. Krim and Sonnabend, the Consumer Treatment Initiative would "seek out promising interventions to prevent progression to full-blown AIDS in those at risk; design experimental treatment protocols for the controlled trial of such interventions; and implement these trials in human volunteer subjects who are at risk for the development of AIDS." The Consumer Treatment Initiative (CTI), a National Institutes of Health in miniature, was to establish an Institutional Review Board to review protocols in accordance with federal regulations governing human subject experimentation. It would organize, too, a scientific and medical committee to seek out, suggest and evaluate promising interventions. It aimed at assembling for clinical trials 1,000 individuals with lymphadenopathy and abnormalities in immunologic evaluation and 500 who were symptomatic with, for example, weight loss, thrush (an opportunistic disease associated with HIV infection that causes lesions in the mouth), fevers and diarrhea. A fundraising goal of $25,000 was proposed for an initial six-month budget. The new committee was to solicit the sponsorship of drug companies with products available for testing.

Its cooperation rejected by CDC, the AIDS community was embarking on its own program of research, seeking collaboration with major pharmaceutical companies and mobilizing the HIV-infected community and physicians with large rosters of HIV patients in a united effort to advance the fight against the virus. It was to be hoped that CTI (subsequently the Community Research Initiative [CRI]) would develop nonbureaucratic procedures that might offer models for improving efficiency in similar huge government agencies.

Michael Callen was appointed as contact person for the new initiative. Lanky but seemingly in perfect health, with an alternating grave and ironic manner, Michael was one of the first individuals in the United States to be diagnosed with AIDS, or rather with "GRID" (Gay Related Immune Deficiency), the original name of the syndrome. In 1977, developing a high fever in conjunction with bloody diarrhea, Michael collapsed in his apartment. At the Gay Clinic, Dr. Sonnabend was recommended as a physician. ("Luck of the draw!" Michael exclaims.) Sonnabend included Michael's blood sample among ten that he sent to a colleague at the University of Nebraska for analysis. The test showed that Michael was seriously immune compromised. In the summer of 1982 he was diagnosed as having cryptosporidiosis, a parasite previously found only in livestock and an opportunistic disease associated with AIDS.

The diagnosis was "a cosmic kick in the butt."

"Some claim," Michael said, "that because I am not dead after these five years I was misdiagnosed and never had AIDS. In fact, I have been hospitalized about six times and have had innumerable transfusions. About ten percent of us PWAs have survived after five years. Many people after four years or so no longer even identify themselves as PWAs, for the stress is difficult to endure. There comes a time of burnout."

How did Michael account for his survival as one of the 10 percent and as one of those not suffering from burnout? "Prophylaxis, luck and the love of a good man," said Michael. "I met my lover the week of my diagnosis." (Dr. Sonnabend was one of the first physicians to prescribe bactrim as a prophylaxis against a recurrence of PCP—pneumocystis carinii pneumonia—one of the most common and most dangerous of the opportunistic diseases affecting PWAs.)

"Having the right attitude won't guarantee that you live a long time," Michael noted, "but having the wrong attitude will pretty much guarantee that you will go quickly." In a book of PWA experiences he edited, *Surviving and Thriving with AIDS—Hints for the Newly Diagnosed*, Michael summed up the philosophy that by 1986 more and more PWAs were beginning to adopt: "AIDS need not be a death sentence. I am living proof that not everyone dies from AIDS. . . . However long you have to live . . . you should live your life to the fullest."

With Sonnabend and Krim, Michael had been one of the founders of the AIDS Medical Foundation, the forerunner to the American Foundation for AIDS Research (AmFAR), which became the leading AIDS research foundation in the nation. A founder also of the PWA Coalition, he became editor of the Coalition newsletter, the "PWA Newsline," a fifty-page monthly with a circulation of 7,500. With Sonnabend, Michael and another PWA wrote a pamphlet entitled, "How to Have Sex in an Epidemic," the first safer sex publication in New York.

"We Need Not Die!": Michael May and the Israeli Therapy

On February 24, 1987 the New York PWA Coalition held a public forum on "Alternative Treatments for AIDS." Although many, perhaps most, of the 400 people crowding into the barnlike ground floor of the Gay and Lesbian Community Center on West 13th Street were PWAs or PWARCs (Persons with AIDS Related Complex), the atmosphere in the hall was of heady expectation, inspired both by the topic for discussion and by the assemblage of so many people with a common purpose.

Two physicians who spoke about promising drugs as yet unauthorized by FDA were listened to with respectful attention, but it was Michael May whom people had come to hear. Everyone present knew his name, for over the previous four months he had told his story repeatedly in television interviews and to the press. No other report of an AIDS treatment had stirred such hope.

A few weeks earlier John James, editor of *AIDS Treatment News*, had published a letter from Michael in which Michael related his experiences during the previous year and a half. Michael wrote:

> I noticed a difficulty with my health during the summer of 1985. . . . My energy dropped. . . . During the fall I suffered with strange illnesses: an ear infection that wouldn't respond to antibiotics; athlete's foot; frequent colds. In January of 1986 I had the worst "flu" of my life, and it wouldn't go away. Toward the end of the month I developed a tightness in my chest and a bad cough. . . . The ELISA test, a T-lymphocyte subset and a viral culture confirmed what I did not want to hear. AIDS. I was given bactrim for the pneumocystis and the cough abated, but my strength was gone. I could no longer work. During February and March, I developed painful sores. A fungus spread to my legs and arms. My skin was scaly, with red blotches. I had fits of perspiration at night. I had fevers. I couldn't eat. I became thin. Worst of all was the generalized feeling through my body that I was dying. Indeed, I was dying.

Of average height and of indeterminate age (he was actually 40), bespectacled and of unprepossessing features, Michael recounted to his audience how upon his diagnosis he invited his mother to his home to inform her of the bad news. "You can't die," she declared firmly. "Who will take care of me in my old age?" Her remark was not meant to be unkind. Indeed, she immediately wrote for advice to a friend, an American Israeli who was doing graduate work at the Weizmann Institute. The friend brought the problem to Meir Shinitzky, one of the leading scientists at the world-renowned institute and the developer of a particular formula for egg lecithin called Active Lipid 721. (A lipid is a fatty component of a cell, and the three components of this lecithin were in a proportion of 7:2:1.) This variant of a common health-food product had shown promise in a clinical study of geriatric patients with immune deficiency.

At the time Shinitzky was conducting experiments with geriatric patients Robert Gallo of the National Cancer Institute described the AIDS virus as having an envelope with an extraordinarily high ratio of one to six between cholesterol and lipids. When

Shinitzky's work in reducing cholesterol in membranes through AL721 was brought to Gallo's attention, he and his colleagues made an in vitro experiment of AL721 with the AIDS virus. In November 1985 in a letter to the prestigious *New England Journal of Medicine*, these scientists declared, "AL721 is a promising new candidate for clinical investigation in the treatment of AIDS and AIDS-related complex."

Interviewed upon the appearance of the letter, Fulton Crews of the School of Medicine of the University of Florida at Gainesville, one of the signatories, explained the mode of operation of the lecithin compound: "Cholesterol makes membranes rigid and hard. So when you pull the cholesterol out, the membrane does, in essence, melt. . . . This membrane engineering may provide a whole new therapeutic approach in a large variety of viruses." Another signatory, P. S. Sarin of the Institute for Cancer Research, stated that although he believed AL721 would kill the virus produced by virus-producing cells and was itself nontoxic, he thought it would be premature to call it a cure.

(As far as the signers of that letter or the Israeli researchers were aware, this variant of egg lecithin had never been used to treat an individual with AIDS. In fact, a test had been made a year earlier, in 1984, but that information, as we shall see, had been suppressed by the American firm that had obtained from the Weizmann Institute the universal license for the manufacture and distribution of AL721.)

Upon reading the Gallo letter, Shinitzky said to Yehuda Skornik, a surgeon at Rokach Hospital in Tel Aviv with whom Shinitzky had been engaged in cancer research, "Let's try it with a patient."

In March 1986, five months after the appearance of the Gallo letter, Michael May's Israeli friend called Shinitzky. Shinitzky asked Skornik, "Are you ready?"

"If you want me to do it, let's start," was Skornik's reply.

One day, Michael told the audience at the PWA Coalition meeting, he received by express mail "a most remarkable document—a letter full of promise." By that time, he recounted, "my condition had deteriorated to the point where I had hardly strength to breathe. I knew my death was imminent." His mother Shirley and his lover carried him in a wheelchair onto a plane. The next day, with his mother and his lover supporting him under the arms, Michael climbed the steps of Rokach Hospital to Dr. Yehuda Skornik's office.

Skornik relates that Michael was unable to sit up on the couch, and he seemed at the point of fainting. After a brief examination, the groggy Michael heard Skornik say, "Don't worry, we'll soon have you up and about."

That first day and during the following two weeks Skornik administered a daily dose of ten grams of AL721 orally, a dosage based on Shinitzky's experience with geriatric patients and in conformity with the physiology of the human cells to be treated. Noticing no change in his condition after a week, Michael discussed burial arrangements with his mother and his lover. After ten days his condition was still unchanged. One day, after two weeks, however, he called Skornik: "I feel stronger," he announced. "My diarrhea is better. I'm eating again." Skornik jumped into his car and drove to the hotel.

Michael was up and about and seemingly full of energy.

"It's working!" Michael exclaimed.

"Don't draw any conclusions," warned Skornik, incredulous at the extraordinary transformation. "It's too soon to be certain."

After three weeks Michael boarded a plane for the United States, this time without a wheelchair and without support, walking on his own.

Fearing an unfavorable reaction in the scientific community to a premature announcement of the effectiveness of AL721 in the treatment of AIDS, Skornik asked Michael not to publicize his experience. Upon his return, however, Michael's friends remarked upon his extraordinary improvement. He persuaded eight PWA acquaintances to travel to Israel for treatment. Word reached the press. In October 1986 Michael was interviewed on television.

At the PWA Coalition meeting on the evening of February 24, 1987 the audience saw a man seemingly in perfect health, walking vigorously and speaking in a strong though quiet voice. "I have no more physical symptoms," Michael declared. "The infections have gone; the night sweats have stopped; I have no more fevers. I am able to eat again, and my weight is close to normal. The last symptoms to disappear were the red blotches and scaling on my face. In October these, too, went away. I do remain easily excitable," he admitted. "When you have been to Auschwitz and survived, I think you never get over it."

Michael spread a small quantity of AL721 on two slices of bread. (It resembled butter in appearance and consistency.) This was the dose he took every morning, he explained. He invited people from the audience to come to the platform to taste it. Two men came forward and ate the slices of bread.

This was all there was to it?

Michael's recovery was due to such a simple treatment?

Michael was obviously pleased with the audience's response. He was unaware, however, that upon returning to their seats, the two volunteer tasters exclaimed to each other, "It has too strong a taste of acetone."

A medical student named Suzanne Phillips[1] turned and asked, "Do you know anything about this substance?"

"We've been making it ourselves," one of the men replied.

There was no opportunity to continue a conversation, for Michael's talk had roused an intense response. There were cries from different parts of the hall: "How can we arrange for treatment in Israel?"

"You can't," replied Michael.

"Why not?"

"The Israelis are unable to treat any more American patients," Michael declared. A murmur of indignation arose. "Why is that?" people shouted.

It simply wasn't possible, Michael insisted.

Several people stood up and demanded a forthright explanation.

Michael would say no more.

---

[1] Suzanne Phillips subsequently received her degree as an M.D. and in 1990 was on the staff at Brooklyn Hospital.

"What are we to do?"

"Why should we be denied?"

The despair in the audience was palpable. More than despair—rancor at yet another incomprehensible obstacle to a possible solution to the horrendous disease, at further frustration in the search for an end to anxiety, fear and pain; to the unremitting cycle of heavy sweats and swollen lymph glands, of bouts with opportunistic diseases one upon another, of checking in and out of hospitals with an exotic variety of pneumonia, with Kaposi's sarcoma, spinal meningitis or a painful eye infection along with a slow deterioration of part of the brain leading to loss of memory and concentration; and a slow wasting away, a decline in energy, a catastrophic loss of weight—until the sufferers with their yellow pallor, sunken cheeks, hollowed eyes and skin stretched so taut as to outline their skulls resembled the miserable creatures liberated from Nazi concentration camps.

One of the men who had run up to the platform to taste the AL721 stood up. He identified himself as James Perez. It was not difficult to make AL721 in your own kitchen, he declared. He had, he admitted, some training in chemistry, but anyone prepared to undertake an uncomplicated but tedious operation, exercising some care, could learn how to make it.

When the meeting broke up, the audience, which had assembled in the expectation of gaining encouragement, departed confused and disgruntled. A crowd pressed about Perez. The medical student Suzanne Phillips joined the group. While doing volunteer work at the Spellman Center for Persons with AIDS at St. Clare's Hospital in Manhattan, she had befriended a PWA. He was wasting away, and it appeared that he had only weeks to live. AL721 might prove his salvation, she thought, as it had proved Michael's.

Perez answered each of his questioners calmly. He gave Suzanne his telephone number. A man who overheard the conversation introduced himself. He was Ron Monroe. He had, he said, a copy of the Israeli patent application, which contained detailed information about AL721. Although he had been thinking of making AL721 in his own apartment, he had hesitated because of his weak background in chemistry. He offered to drop the patent document off at Suzanne's apartment the next day.

◆ ◆ ◆

Interviewed some days after the February meeting, Michael May proved hardly reticent, indeed eager to relate details of a dire conspiracy. An official of the Department of Health and Human Services, according to Michael's sources (which he refused to reveal), had visited Israel and had pressured the Weizmann Institute into dismissing Meir Shinitzky, the developer of AL721. In disgust, Skornik was emigrating from Israel (to a country which Michael declared he was not at liberty to name).

How did Michael account for this U.S. pressure?

Fear of AL721 competition, he replied, for the officially favored therapy AZT.

Michael's tale of conspiracy provided the impetus to the writing of this book.

CHAPTER

"The Israeli Conspiracy"

In April 1987, four months after the meeting at which Michael May related his story, Yehuda Skornik was badgered by some of his colleagues at an international cancer conference at Nice.

(Skornik had not emigrated from Israel at all! He had merely traveled to France to participate in a scientific conference. So much for this portion of Michael May's "conspiracy!")

"How dare you use a treatment," exclaimed a physician from San Francisco with considerable practice among AIDS patients, "that has not undergone standard clinical testing, a double-blind study? How dare you publicize tentative results and offer false hopes to thousands of people suffering from this dreadful epidemic?"

Instilled with the traditional ideal of *rakhmonas* (compassion for the suffering of a fellow human being), a fundamental Hebraic principle in the practice of medicine, Skornik, a religious Jew, matched the indignation of his critic with equal passion, berating the entire assemblage: "Compare the uproar against me to the silence at this doctor's report of eleven deaths [among his AIDS patients]. . . . I start with a treatment known to be nontoxic, and you claim that I am a murderer." Turning directly toward the physician from San Francisco, Skornik challenged him. "All of my patients have survived and shown improvement," he declared. "How many patients have you saved? As to your demand for a double-blind study before application of this treatment," he continued, "there has been such a study—on the one hand, the thousands of patients never treated with AL721 who have died and, on the other, the dozens who have been so treated and have so far survived."

In this exchange was mirrored a struggle splitting the medical community, between those (including some Israeli physicians) who insisted upon the maintenance of established clinical testing procedures even during a medical crisis like the current AIDS epidemic and those who, like the organizers of the New York Consumer Treatment Initiative, proclaimed that flexibility was required in such an emergency.

◆ ◆ ◆

At the Weizmann Institute is Shinitzky's laboratory, in the basement of the Ullman building, at the end of a long corridor half-blocked by machinery and supplies. It is a cramped L-shaped area with the larger rectangular portion some fifteen by ten feet in area with a window at ground level.

(Shinitzky had not been dismissed from his post at the Weizmann Institute, nor had any U.S. official ever suggested his dismissal. So much for this second aspect of Michael May's conspiracy!)

On a table along one wall of Shinitzky's laboratory stood a crude iron mechanism with a pair of globes in which a yellow liquid rose and fell in a constant slow rhythm, a primitive device that might have been borrowed from an exhibit of eighteenth-century mechanics in the Smithsonian Institution. In the adjoining office, about the size of a closet kitchenette in a New York studio apartment, the desk was cluttered with documents.

Shinitzky is less than average height, frank and trusting, with the wry and slightly cynical air of a naif who had been gulled too often. As a youth he had been uncertain whether to become a scientist or a violinist. (On the wall of his laboratory hangs an autographed picture of Toscanini.)

After obtaining his doctorate at the Weizmann Institute, winning the most prestigious university award in Israel, the J. F. Kennedy Prize, Shinitzky did postdoctoral work at the University of Illinois at Urbana. Upon returning to Israel, Shinitzky was certain of the field in which he wished to specialize—biological membranes, a virgin territory of significance in many diseases. With a machine he constructed for studying membranes, he achieved a worldwide reputation. In the seventies Shinitzky came across a study done at the University of Virginia showing that VSV, an envelope virus that infects horses, contains a high percentage of cholesterol in the membrane. When the cholesterol was reduced in vitro, the virus lost its infectivity and became dormant. With the reintroduction of cholesterol, the virus regained its infectivity.

In a two-volume work he edited and published in 1984 entitled *Physiology of Membrane Fluidity*, Shinitzky observed:

> The obvious candidate for membrane fluidization both in vitro and in vivo [with living subjects] is lecithin from natural sources (e.g., egg yolk), which can fluidize membranes either by extracting excess cholesterol or by incorporation into the membrane. . . . Recently we developed in our laboratory a potent lipid mixture, designated as Active Lipid (AL), for membrane fluidization. . . . This mixture is composed of about 70 per cent neutral glycerides, 20 per cent lecithin and 10 per cent phosphatidyl ethanolamine, all from hen egg yolk. [Thus the name AL721!]

◆ ◆ ◆

In 1979, on a plane from a geriatrics conference in Brussels, Shinitzky and David Samuel, another Weizmann Institute scientist, discussed their research projects and realized that they could collaborate effectively. Samuel, the son of the second Viscount Samuel, governor of Palestine under the British mandate after World War I, was born and educated in Palestine. After serving in Burma during World War II and as administrator for Sumatra after the war, he obtained a degree in chemistry at Oxford and then became one of the first graduate students at the Weizmann Institute. Subsequently he did postdoctoral work at Harvard and at Berkeley.

Shinitzky was experimenting with lipids in relation to the immune system of the aged, and Samuel was studying the effects of aging on the brain. Under their supervision, a graduate student named David Heron discovered that injections of AL721 in animals brought a reversal in the stiffening and an increase in the cholesterol count of brain membranes, changes associated with the aging process as well as with drug addiction and alcoholism. In a report of their findings Heron, Shinitzky and Samuel declared, "These results could be the basis for a novel innocuous treatment which may facilitate the rehabilitation of drug and alcohol addicts."

This study was followed by another conducted by graduate student Mark Lyte, who had come to the Institute from the University of Virginia. In January 1984 at a conference on aging at Zurich, Shinitzky and Lyte reported: "Active Lipid diet was found to markedly improve immune competence of the aged, and it is likely that in parallel it elicits a significant restoration of brain functions. . . . [The agent for the] restoration of impaired membrane fluidity . . . should freely cross the blood-brain barrier and should exert its effect before being metabolized by the liver." Ordinary lecithin, unable to cross the blood-brain barrier, was blocked from access to brain membranes, but AL, a variant of egg lecithin, did have this capacity. "Inasmuch as AL," the researchers observed in addition, "is a par excellence nutrient, no adverse reactions could be expected when given to men."

A three-week clinical test was conducted with sixteen people over 75 years of age, all immune-suppressed. "After several days of AL diet," according to Shinitzky, "a significant increase in response to mitogens[1] was observed. After about three weeks the patients' immune systems reached a level typical of that in young people. Upon cessation of the diet the lymphocyte responsiveness slowly declined towards the initial basal level."

"Within weeks," recounted Yehuda Skornik, who had followed the experiment, "the patients experienced a general sense of well being; they were clearer in their thinking, some of them stopped smoking; one of them had an improvement in his sex life. Not only was there a change in the T cells with the entire group, but also in

---

[1] A substance that causes lymphocytes, the blood-borne cells that produce antibodies or are otherwise involved in immune responses, to proliferate.

the responsiveness of those T cells. In one case there was a reduction of cholesterol levels in the blood—a change that suggested other directions for future research."

Working with Shinitzky was his laboratory assistant, Rachel Haimovich, an attractive, modest, dark-haired woman in her early thirties. (David Samuel insisted that "there have been really just three of us involved in the AL721 investigation, Meir and I and Rachel Haimovich.") In June 1987 Rachel Haimovich could often be found standing with an oar-like instrument over a metal container about half the size of a gasoline drum churning a yellow batter. The crude iron mechanism with glass globes on the laboratory table along with Rachel and her churn supplied AL721 for AIDS patients in Israel as well as small quantities for overseas researchers and physicians and for patients previously treated in Israel.

"This devoted young woman," Shinitzky recounted, "tells me that she can't sleep at night. She thinks that every minute she is not mixing the AL721 people may be dying for the lack of it."

The limitation on Israeli production of AL721 was stipulated by the American licensee for AL721, James Jacobson, Jr., who feared both litigation in the event a patient in Israel suffered harm from treatment with the substance and complications with the Food and Drug Administration in authorization of AL721 as an ethical pharmaceutical (a drug available only by prescription). Jacobson permitted the Israelis to produce and to prescribe AL721 only if no compensation was involved. Rachel Haimovich was volunteering her time to prepare the material.

Shinitzky and Samuel were cautious in commenting on their relationship with the American licensee. Whenever disagreements arose, Jacobson threatened the Israelis with legal action through his uncle and partner, Leslie Jacobson, a member of a distinguished New York law firm of which one of the partners was Sargent Shriver, a brother-in-law of the Kennedys. The Israelis had no desire to be diverted from their research by involvement in litigation.

The Israeli Physicians
YEHUDA SKORNIK

Following upon Michael May's disclosure of his Israeli experience, Skornik received a flood of telephone calls. Dependent upon the AL721 Rachel Haimovich produced in her free time in Shinitzky's laboratory and bearing a full schedule as a practicing surgeon, Skornik was restricted as to the number of patients he could treat. Rarely did he return home before midnight or arrive at the hospital later than seven in the morning. On the other hand, he found it difficult to refuse any request for help. "I'm a doctor," Shinitzky quoted Skornik as saying, "and I cannot see people dying. If an AIDS patient comes here, I will give him this material."

Skornik's first overseas appeal came in December 1986, some nine months after his experience with Michael May. It came from the brother of a 31-year-old AIDS patient whose New York physician gave him only weeks to live. When Skornik hesitated to accept another patient, the man himself came to the telephone. Until six years earlier he had been a drug addict, he explained, and now he was paying for the addiction with AIDS. "I would like to live," he said. "I want to get married. I want another chance at a better life." "Okay, come ahead," said Skornik.

The man arrived in a wheelchair accompanied by his father, mother, brother and fiancee along with a supply of all kinds of infusions, hypoalimentations and solutions. Skornik initiated the treatment immediately. Within two weeks a chronic fever disappeared. Since his patient began to eat normally, Skornik was able to remove the hypoalimentation tube.

Six months later, in June 1987, Skornik reported that the man no longer exhibited symptoms of AIDS. All his blood tests had shown significant improvement. "Today," he said, "I received a post card from him in Italy, where he's gone on vacation with his fiancee."

A second request for treatment came from a physician in Alaska in regard to two former drug addicts. The physician enclosed a letter from the couple. The man and his wife had spent all their savings on treatment, to no avail. They were in despair and thinking of suicide. They had read of Michael May's experience. Skornik, they thought, was their last hope.

Two days after the letters arrived, before Skornik had a chance to reply, the couple appeared in Tel Aviv. "What choice did I have?" Skornik exclaimed.

After ten days or so the couple returned to Alaska. Improvement began very quickly. The wife had suffered chronically from herpes. The herpes disappeared. She recovered sufficiently to return to work. The husband, less fortunate, continued to be plagued by opportunistic infections.

"The selection among whom to treat and whom to refuse is very difficult," Skornik admitted. "I don't have any system. . . . All those that we have accepted for treatment have been in a really desperate condition. In one case a man called and said, 'My one son died in a heart operation; the other is about to die of AIDS at the age of 28, will you treat him?' When I said that I would treat him, he was astonished. I could not refuse to treat the only remaining child."

This young man had suffered severe brain damage from the AIDS virus. Two weeks after receiving a quantity of AL721, the mother telephoned to report that her son was lifting his head. After three weeks he began to sit up and to speak, though indistinctly. The following week, when Skornik was passing through New York on his way back from the International AIDS Conference in Washington, the mother called to report that her son had lost consciousness. The visiting nurse said that it would be a waste of effort to take him to a hospital.

Skornik found the man in a small two-room apartment in Brooklyn. His mother had moved in to nurse him. "If he were my son," Skornik told the woman, "I would bring him to a hospital for fluids and electrolysis."

Two weeks later Skornik received word that the man was home from the hospital and improving. He was opening his eyes and watching television. "We don't give up quickly," Skornik insisted.

Skornik had a severely ill patient in Staten Island, a 31-year-old drug addict who was undergoing withdrawal treatment. He, too, had suffered brain damage. When Skornik visited him, he found that with AL721 the man had become stronger. He had regained his appetite. His mother complained, however, that he remembered nothing and would not utter a word. He had been a computer technician. Skornik sat down and asked the man for suggestions about the purchase of a computer. The patient responded rationally and without inhibition.

Skornik instructed the mother not to argue or to discuss her son's condition in front of him. She called some days later to report that he was continuing to improve, and the man himself came to the telephone to speak with Skornik.

"My colleagues ask," Skornik said, "why I accept patients in critical condition. 'They'll die on you and ruin your statistics,' they say. 'If you want to succeed, take lighter cases, you'll get better results.' I always answer, 'I don't care about statistics.' In fact, I get good results even with serious cases."

By June 1987 Skornik had twenty-eight patients under treatment, fourteen from the United States and the others from Italy, Germany, South Africa and England. Israeli patients he turned over to Israel-Yust, head of Immunology at Ikhivod Hospital in Tel Aviv. None of Skornik's patients had suffered any bad side effects from the AL721 other than brief bouts of diarrhea. All showed improvement, including a considerable number of supposedly terminal cases—all, that is, except one. Upon returning to San Francisco, this man had developed a lung infection unrelated to AIDS. The hospital refused to operate on him because of his AIDS, and he died.

At the IInd International Conference on AIDS early in June 1987, in Washington, D.C., a group of Skornik's American patients assembled, without prior organization, to honor Skornik and to support him in championing AL721 as an AIDS therapy. One of the group carried a large sign reading, "AL721, a new lifesaving material from Israel." They distributed leaflets to the delegates. When Skornik saw the group with their sign, he removed the nametag from his jacket and stole into the hall, hoping to escape notice.

A special meeting on AL721 was held in a church across the street from the meeting hall. Skornik was disappointed at the small attendance. "It's true," he admitted, "that we had only 28 patients on whom to report. Even Gallo made no mention of AL721 although he was the one who pointed out its potential against the virus."

Shinitzky quoted one of the other Israelis who attended the conference as saying: "You wouldn't believe how stupid we look in the eyes of the Americans because of AL721. They do not think that this is the way studies should be conducted."

As for clinical testing, Skornik declared, "The proper study is, of course, a blind study. That means, however, readiness to sacrifice AIDS patients either by giving them a placebo or by compelling them to await results before having the opportunity to take advantage of the substance. In double-blind studies with other substances

PWAs have sabotaged the tests by splitting the doses among themselves so that no one was on a placebo. What else can they do?

"I think," said Skornik, "that everyone who is sero-positive should take AL721. The early stage may be the best time to treat those patients. I would test them and then after six months make another test of the T cell count and also of the virus itself. I suspect that in those patients this treatment may result in the elimination of the infection. Their immune systems, which are still strong, may be able to deal with the weakened virus."

ISRAEL YUST

Israel Yust, the physician who assumed the treatment of Skornik's Israeli patients at the Ikhivod Hospital, was born in 1937 of Polish immigrants. He fought in the Sinai campaign in 1956; subsequently, after completing his medical training at the Hebrew University Medical School, he served in a medical unit in the 1967 war and later again in the Sinai. For three years he did postdoctoral work in immunology at the National Institutes of Health in Bethesda. Upon returning to Israel he established an immunology unit at the Ikhivod Hospital.

The Ikhivod Hospital had its first AIDS patient in 1981 or 1982. The doctors did not recognize the illness until the man came down with pneumocystis carinii pneumonia and other opportunistic diseases and finally mycobacterium avian and Kaposi's sarcoma. He died in 1984. A few months before coming to the hospital, this man had donated blood. When a woman who underwent plastic surgery of the breast subsequently died of AIDS, an examination of the records revealed that she had received a transfusion with his blood.

By June 1987 Yust had used AL721 with eleven patients in different stages of AIDS. His evaluation of AL721 was generally favorable. "Above all," he said, "it does no harm. Then, too, most of the AIDS patients have a sense of well-being after something like two weeks. With a chronic disease with ups and downs and with patients taking other medications for opportunistic diseases, it is difficult to assess AL721."

As an example of the need for a double-blind controlled test of AL721, Yust related his experience with a patient referred to him by Skornik. Confined to a wheelchair and deteriorating rapidly, the patient sought treatment with AL721. Yust insisted he first obtain his physician's approval. The physician stated categorically that if the patient took AL721 he would no longer treat him. After giving assurance that he would submit to the doctor's judgment, the patient came to Yust for the AL721 anyhow. He showed rapid improvement and was even able to do without his wheelchair. The original physician decided to administer AZT. After six days in the hospital on doses of AZT, the patient went home. His physician, unaware that his patient had been taking AL721, announced to the press: "AZT helped my patient." The very next day the patient came down with convulsions, often a side effect of AZT.

"Thus you see," said Yust, "how careful you must be about coming to conclusions. If you ask me, I think it was the AL721 that accounted for his improvement. Can I prove it? No!

"When I am asked," said Yust, "whether we should administer AL721 now to AIDS patients, I am not opposed, but I want a double-blind study once and for all. We should try it on people who are merely sero-positive or with ARC [AIDS Related Complex] patients who are not critically ill and see whether they benefit from it. Emotional involvement like Skornik's is all well and good," he continued, "but emotion has no place in scientific testing. We cannot deal simply with estimations and probabilities. A controlled study will expose whether it is useful on its own or whether it should be used in combination with another treatment, perhaps with a lesser dose of AZT than is now prescribed."

ZWI BENTWICH
Zwi Bentwich obtained his medical training at the Medical School of the Hebrew University in Jerusalem, where he is currently a professor. The Kaplan Hospital, in fact, is the teaching hospital for the school. After pursuing postdoctoral work at the Weizmann Institute and the Hebrew University, Bentwich spent two years at Rockefeller University in New York and a year's sabbatical at the University of California at Los Angeles. In his carriage and speech, Bentwich gives the impression of a military man. Indeed, he served in the Israeli air force and then as a surgeon in a helicopter rescue squad.

The first AIDS case at the Kaplan Hospital was flown in from San Francisco in 1982 for treatment with the thymus cumulic factor (an immuno-modulator developed at the Weizmann Institute, purified and synthesized from the thymus gland of calves).

Why had the patient not received this treatment in the United States?

"It was not available there. They had not approved it as a treatment," intervened Shinitzky with asperity.

In any event, the treatment proved ineffective, and the patient died. He had had many contacts in the Israeli gay community, and upon his arrival at the hospital Bentwich and his colleagues with exemplary foresight initiated an intensive investigation of Israeli homosexuals. By the summer of 1987 Bentwich and his associates had tested about 1,000 gays. Through periodic retesting they had followed some of the initial 250 for two years. They discovered that sero-conversion (change from negative to positive in viral infection) was very low in Israel in comparison to the United States—no more than two and a trifle percentage points over a period of three years. Among the entire group of 1,000, not more than 15 percent had become sero-positive after four years. "In the United States, on the other hand," Bentwich noted, "if you start at five per cent, within two years it reaches thirty, forty and even fifty per cent.

"I think Israeli gays have profoundly changed their sexual habits," Bentwich explained. "By the time this change occurred in the United States, it was too late though sero-conversion has started to decline in the United States, too. In Israel we are fortunate in that we started with a low incidence and as a result of timely intervention, we have maintained this low incidence.

"The general theory," said Bentwich, "is that gays are particularly susceptible to the AIDS virus because of the large number of contacts of some of them. I was confident that this was not a sufficient explanation." Indeed, Bentwich found that even homosexuals who are not sero-positive were, as a group, more immune impaired than heterosexuals. "Like IV drug users and hemophiliacs," he declared, "homosexuals who come down with the disease are probably immune impaired prior to infection by the virus."

According to Bentwich, a difference between promiscuous homosexuals and heterosexuals lies in anal intercourse. "If you inject sperm into an animal anywhere but in the vagina," he said, "it suffers immune suppression." In addition, sperm gets into the system more readily through the rectum than through the barriers that usually prevent such penetration. The results from the change in sexual behavior among gays, he noted, support this contention.

"We do not know," he noted, "who or why one gets the disease after being infected. It is clear in any case that continued promiscuity brings a further assault on the immune system."

At the Kaplan Hospital Bentwich had introduced AL721 only three months earlier, in March 1987. He had one patient who responded dramatically after about two weeks on AL721—an IV drug user who had lived in France. Subsequently, however, he suffered a relapse. "His case," Bentwich warned, "provides an example of the need for caution in prematurely assessing results. Nothing," he insisted, "is going to be resolved until we have a long and completely scientific study."

Would Bentwich suggest that the United States with hundreds of patients dying every month await such tests before administering AL721?

No. "I was brought up as a good Jewish boy with a strong prejudice against homosexuals," Bentwich explained, "but when one treats AIDS patients and sees how dreadfully they suffer from this terrible disease, all prejudice evaporates. From the perspective of compassion and from the little scientific knowledge that we have, one can say that there is no harm in using this treatment. It may very well be found that it is effective. Meanwhile, nothing is to be lost. But I also think one should get the most out of clinical trials so that we gain something and don't just do things in the air."

◆ ◆ ◆

In the fall of 1986 Undersecretary of Health Don Newman and Bob Brock, the science attaché of the U.S. Embassy at Tel Aviv, visited Shinitzky at the Weizmann Institute. At the end of their two-hour discussion, Shinitzky asked Newman to inform him upon his return to Washington of any results stemming from this meeting. To his chagrin Shinitzky did not hear a word either from Newman or from Brock.

(This event was the basis for Michael May's report of the visit of an American official to Israel and of the supposed pressure on the Weizmann Institute for

Shinitzky's dismissal! With this final evidence, May's entire "conspiracy" was exposed as mere fantasy.)

According to Brock, before expressing a judgment on AL721 Newman was awaiting further word from Gallo. "If Gallo is delaying in giving a full recommendation," Newman said, "there must be a reason." (Scientists had been waiting for more than a year and a half for a further statement from Gallo.)

In April 1988 in an interview with Phil Zwickler of the *New York Native*, Shinitzky asserted that he was confident that a cure could be found for the HIV epidemic if the United States distributed $1 million to each of a hundred institutions throughout the world, each to do a separate type of research. "I can assure you," Shinitzky declared, "from my own experience, a solution could be found within two to three years."

Phil Zwickler died of AIDS in May 1991.

First PWA Initiatives
with AL721

Throughout the United States PWAs had reached the same conclusion as Dr. Zwi Bentwich in Israel that for people otherwise doomed to early and often horrendous death nothing was to be lost in experimenting with any treatments that offered even the slightest hope of benefit. Persuaded that they could not rely upon governmental officials to make such therapies available, AIDS activists resolved they would have to assume that responsibility themselves.

Unknown to most of the audience at the February 1987 meeting at which Michael May caused such a sensation, a group of PWAs in New York were already making plans for distributing AL721 or an AL721 analog. Early in January Tom Hannan called a meeting in his Greenwich Village apartment to discuss action for making available promising drugs that were awaiting FDA approval.

Tom had good reason to be searching for an AIDS therapy. Tom's "life partner" Steve Roach, a chemist at Columbia University, had symptoms of a grave disorder as early as 1978 and repeated bouts of PCP (pneumocystis carinii pneumonia) since his diagnosis as a PWA in 1984.

Below average height, with dark, thinning hair and an attractive, guileless face, Tom exuded warmth and zest. In 1976, when he was 25, Tom met Steve, and they remained together except for interludes when Tom traveled back and forth to Europe to pursue his career as a singer. After Steve came down with PCP and was, accordingly, diagnosed as having full-blown AIDS, Tom remained in New York.

Late in 1986 Tom, too, came down with PCP. His physician put him on bactrim. "It was a horror story," Tom said. "Between the lung condition and the bactrim, my fever remained at 104 continuously for four weeks." His doctor finally switched him to a new prophylaxis, aerosolized pentamedine, a spray without bad side effects.

The PWAs who responded to Tom's invitation to that January meeting were impelled to action not only by the general awakening of militancy in the gay community and by an intense frustration at incompetence and indifference at all levels of government but also by an emerging hope that HIV infection did not necessarily signify a swift death sentence, a hope inspired in part by FDA and NIH's touting of AZT as a therapy that at least delayed the progress of the disease. On the other hand, in the fall of 1986 and the early months of 1987, only PWAs who had been afflicted with PCP were able to obtain AZT. All others faced an indefinite and possibly fatal delay. In addition, reports of serious side effects and even of the demise of participants in AZT trials as well as uncertainty about the longer-range effects of the drug made many of those infected with HIV hesitant to try it.

Furthermore, with the widespread suspicion of governmental agencies within the AIDS community, many PWAs mistrusted official claims for AZT and the exclusive emphasis on AZT in government-funded research projects. They were, in addition, angry at what they considered profiteering on suffering by the Burroughs Wellcome corporation. Leading activist Michael Callen even advised against taking AZT altogether.

With the PWA Coalition's Consumer Treatment Initiative still in a planning stage, the small group that assembled at Tom's apartment reasoned that there was at least a temporary role for a committee in which PWAs and other HIV-positive individuals might plan initiatives on their own in an Ad Hoc Committee for a Community Research Initiative.

With the many rapid changes in the AIDS scene since 1987, people who have remained active in the AIDS community may have forgotten the enormous impact of AL721 as an AIDS therapy in that year and the following year. Although in 1992 hundreds still maintained their trust in the efficacy of AL721, they no longer represented a major segment of the PWA community, and AL721 had long been ignored by the media. In 1987, however, of the numerous therapies tested by people with the HIV infection, AL721, for a series of reasons, represented a natural first choice for community distribution.

1. Since AL721 was merely a variant of lecithin, long an over-the-counter health-food product, PWA distributors had little fear of FDA police action as they would have had in making available drugs awaiting FDA approval.
2. Robert C. Gallo, the co-discoverer of HIV and an unflagging promoter of AZT, along with other U.S. scientists, had announced that in in vitro trials AL721 had proved effective against HIV.
3. Unlike other underground therapies, AL721 was backed by the prestige of a world-renowned research institution, the Weizmann Institute. (Indeed, the institute suddenly achieved a popular renown it had never previously enjoyed.) Furthermore, PWAs were reassured by the easy accessibility of both Shinitzky and Skornik, who responded to letters and telephone calls with patience and compassion. Their generosity contrasted sharply with the bureaucratic indifference and arrogance often encountered among U.S. health service officials.

4. Whereas the single therapy authorized by FDA was the most costly drug ever produced for mass distribution, AL721 was not only comparatively inexpensive but also possible to produce at minimal cost in private kitchens.

5. The publicity accorded Michael May's successful experience with AL721 had evoked an extraordinary emotional response in the AIDS community, especially in face of the conflicting reports regarding side effects and other drawbacks of AZT. AL721 became in a sense the community's own therapy against the government-sponsored, multinational corporation–controlled, profit-oriented AZT.

Invited to serve as medical consultant to the new committee formed at Tom Hannan's apartment, Dr. Joe Sonnabend accepted with enthusiasm. "The objective," as he saw it, "was to get AL721 to the people who needed it. I had the view that in the case of AIDS in dealing with non-toxic treatments we don't have to be hostages to completion of clinical trials. In an urgent situation, it is unethical to withhold anything that can possibly be beneficial. This seems to be a novel thought to our new breed of scientists. It wouldn't have been novel to their teachers in the fifties."

On January 19 the committee, now much increased in membership, drafted proposals for possible action. "Perhaps naively," Tom later admitted, the group, acting upon a suggestion from Sonnabend, decided first of all to ask Mathilde Krim to convey the group's appeal to Praxis, the company licensed by the Israelis to manufacture and distribute AL721, to release AL721 immediately as a food derivative instead of waiting several years for its approval as a drug by the FDA.

(In the hectic weeks that followed, no one in the committee checked whether Dr. Krim acted upon their request. Some months later, in August, Krim stated privately that she had called James Jacobson, Jr., the founder of Praxis. Jacobson offered to consider the appeal from the ad hoc committee, but in a subsequent telephone conversation he informed Krim that he and his fellow directors in the company were determined to press for FDA authorization of AL721 as a medication and not to release it in advance as a food supplement.)

Other proposals called for (1) producing AL721 in some small laboratory; (2) approaching a congressman to sponsor legislation exempting AL721 from FDA restrictions in the treatment of HIV infection, a measure that might encourage Praxis to release the substance immediately as a food derivative; (3) challenging the AL721 patent; (4) purchasing Praxis stock and mobilizing a shareholders' effort to change Praxis policy; and (5) encouraging reporters to investigate rumors of inside trading at Praxis. "Anything to get Praxis off its ass," commented Tom Hannan.

Within weeks all of these proposals were to be exposed as naive and unrealistic.

At a meeting on January 31 an employee of Bell Laboratories provided a detailed formula for producing AL721. His estimate of the production cost alarmed the group. Steve Gavin, another member of the committee, on the other hand, had purchased an egg lecithin product from a chemical firm at a cost of $134 per half-kilo (approximately one and a half months' supply), a moderate price in comparison with that of AZT, which was then selling for about $800 for a month's supply. The distributor, however, insisted that Gavin sign a document stating that the product would never enter the human food chain, a stipulation that raised questions as to the quality of the product. Both Tom's lover Steve Roach and Steve Gavin presented formulas for producing analogs to AL721 with soy lecithin, less expensive and more readily available than egg lecithin. There was no certainty, of course, that soy lecithin would be equally as effective.

In its January 30 issue *The Sentinel*, a gay newspaper on the West Coast, published instructions for producing AL721, and John James printed the "home formula" in his *AIDS Treatment News*. When Roach assured the group that home production of AL721 did not require advanced scientific training, Jim Perez volunteered to experiment in producing it in his apartment. His friend Kevin Imbusch agreed to work with him. (These were the men who three weeks later at the February 24 meeting ran up to the platform to taste Michael May's samples.)

Born in Texas of Mexican-American parents, Jim had come north to complete his education and was about to obtain a master of science degree. A year earlier, at the age of 33, he had come down with Kaposi's sarcoma and had developed lesions externally over his entire body as well as internally, in his pulmonary tract and intestines. He suffered excruciating pain.

After two decades in the United States Kevin, a man in his fifties, still retained a heavy Scottish brogue. At a PWA discussion group meeting in September 1986 he and Jim went out together during the luncheon break. At the restaurant Jim began to perspire so profusely that his shirt was quickly drenched. "Will you stay with me," he asked Kevin, "until we go back to the meeting?"

Some weeks later Kevin sent Jim a photocopy of an article appearing in the gay weekly *The New York Native* about Michael May's experience with AL721. (Kevin also sent a copy to Joe Sonnabend, who for several years had been his physician.) Jim called and said, "We ought to look into this."

When at Tom's apartment the man who worked at Bell Laboratories distributed a sheet of directions for making AL721, Jim assured Kevin that the procedure was as easy as baking a cake. At a local supermarket they bought ten dozen eggs and at a chemical supply house, two gallons of acetone, a vitamin E solution and two other chemicals. In Jim's tiny kitchen they started making the egg lecithin variant, taking care not to start an explosion with the highly flammable acetone. They placed the material in the freezer, and the next day they took the subway to Canal Street to buy a vacuum pump. After vacuuming, "lo and behold," said Kevin, "there it was!"

Tom and Jim submitted the egg lecithin Steve Gavin had bought and Jim's home product to Arnold S. Lippa, the president of Praxis, for testing at Lippa's laboratory at the City University of New York. To check the accuracy of the analysis, they added six other samples they knew to be totally unsatisfactory. Indeed, Lippa reported that only two of the samples resembled AL721. One, Jim's product, emerged as a close analog. (In future months, the testing of these eight samples would be exploited in a misleading fashion by Praxis.)

"Lippa probably took a liking to Jim," recalled Kevin. "He saw how ill Jim was and said, 'You keep taking this, young man, it is probably your only hope.'"

Kevin was not sure what was the "funny element in Jim's nature" that drew people to him so quickly. "He was shy, almost retiring, but if you got him worked up, he was like a dynamo." The first time Jim came to Kevin's apartment he saw a song by Schubert on the piano, *An die Musik*. Jim asked Kevin to play it. "As soon as I started," Kevin recalled, "he began to sing it in German." A Mormon, Jim had spent some years as a missionary. Subsequently, he had sung at St. Patrick's Cathedral in New York.

Jim and Kevin met about twice a week to make the egg lecithin. By the time Suzanne Phillips, the medical student who had met Jim at the February 24 Michael May meeting, climbed the five flights to Jim's East Harlem apartment for her lesson in making AL721, Jim had become adept at the process. He was often so weak, however, that he had to teach her from his bed. Sometimes when the two of them went shopping for supplies, Jim had to rest at every street corner.

After gaining experience with the process, Suzanne undertook to supply Jim with the lecithin when he was too ill to make it. The two of them taught Ron Monroe, the man who at the February meeting had offered Suzanne his copy of the AL721 patent document, and Ron began making the material in his apartment. Jim, Kevin, Suzanne, Ron and Ron's lover formed a network to help each other and to teach others. Suzanne taught the process to her boyfriend, whose brother had died of AIDS in the spring of 1986. He, too, became involved in the production.

◆ ◆ ◆

Hector Munoz, a 55-year-old psychologist born in Argentina and educated first in Cuba and then at New York University, also had a pressing reason for participating in the ad hoc committee. Three years earlier, shortly after returning to his native Denmark, Hector's lover of nine years wrote that he had come down with AIDS.

A year earlier Hector himself had come down with Kaposi's sarcoma. One of his colleagues at work, also a PWA, advised Hector to stop working. "I wish I had the strength that I have used up by sticking to my job," the colleague said, and on January 16, 1986, the very day the doctor informed him that he had AIDS, Hector quit his job as a dance therapist at the Bronx Psychiatric Hospital. Like Michael Callen, Hector was convinced that much depends upon one's psychological attitude in resisting the virus. "I keep in good balance," he reported, "with food, sleep and exercise, brain and body, all in harmony. It is necessary not to let the disease take over one's life, focusing on others rather than on one's self."

Hector was sensitive to the particular problems faced by Hispanic PWAs. Homosexuals, he noted, confront intense prejudice in the Hispanic community and even in their own families. Their isolation is often intensified by language difficulties and by their ignorance of available public health services. The Gay Men's Health Crisis called upon Hector to assist in counseling Hispanic PWAs, and the PWA Coalition asked him to lead a rap group.

Hector avoided medication except during bouts with opportunistic diseases. Upon reading about AL721 in the *PWA Newsline*, however, he decided that if he would take any medication it would be AL721, a natural substance without side effects.

PWAs Distribute Egg Lecithin

The research organization proposed by the PWA Coalition and promoted by two PWAs and Drs. Sonnabend and Krim was officially established under the name "Community Research Initiative." Tom Hannan was appointed acting administrator. The ad hoc committee Hannan had been instrumental in organizing two months earlier changed its name to the PWA Health Group, with Hannan and Michael Callen as its leaders. Despairing of prompt action by Praxis, the licensee for AL721, the PWA Health Group voted to seek out another company to manufacture the egg lecithin variant for general distribution.

Tom Hannan and Steve Gavin telephoned health-food, vitamin and other firms with possible facilities for manufacturing an AL721 analog. Most firms were frightened off at the mention of the Praxis license for the manufacture and distribution of AL721. After precisely seventeen telephone calls, however, the two men came upon the American Roland Company, a firm in nearby Long Island that had been manufacturing egg lecithin for many years in a plant in Japan. After lengthy negotiations by the PWA Health Group's lawyer, the president of the company agreed to take back and rework any batches that did not meet the 7:2:1 specifications. Upon prepayment at $165 per kilo, the company contracted to supply a hundred kilos for an initial distribution.

Inexperienced as businessmen and wary of being accused of profiteering, Tom Hannan and Michael Callen would have distributed the substance at cost if Michael Hirsch, the director of the PWA Coalition, had not advised them to set a price that would cover the committee's expenses. Accordingly, the PWA Health Group published an announcement that it would supply a kilo of the egg lecithin variant, a three-months' supply, to anyone who sent in a check for $200.

The group advertised their product as egg lecithin and not as AL721, the trademark patented by Praxis, and in their publicity they made no medical claims for their "food supplement." "We probably go overboard," admitted Michael Callen, "in making no medical claims and in saying that there isn't any hard data on the effectiveness of the substance that we're aware of. We come within an inch of discouraging people from getting it because we feel that it's our responsibility not to make unfounded claims."

An immediate problem was to find a hall for the distribution. The Gay and Lesbian Community Center on West 13th Street seemed suitable, but there were possible legal questions involved in the distribution, and the director of the center was hesitant about providing space. Someone suggested seeking a sympathetic church, and after subjecting Tom and Michael to searching questions about their purposes, the Reverend Howard R. Moody and program director Arlene Carmen of Judson Memorial Church on Washington Square offered the use of a rectory hall.

When the American Roland Company failed to meet the promised distribution deadline, "people began to think," said Michael, "that we had gone off to Brazil with the $20,000 we had collected." With the resolution of production problems, however, people who had sent checks for $200 were notified that a distribution of egg lecithin would be held on April 24.

Michael made a videotape portraying himself as Julia Child, the well-known "French Chef" television personality, and gave directions for dividing and mixing the substance.

During the hectic days just before the distribution, Michael said that anyone speaking to Tom on the telephone would have the impression that Tom was on "speed." His phone was ringing day and night, people calling from all over the country about the lecithin distribution. The excitement was especially difficult for Tom's lover. Steve's T4 helper cell count was dangerously low. He had a Kaposi's sarcoma lesion in his mouth that was out of control. The doctor had put him on chemotherapy. He was coming down with PCP for the third time.

Tom was uncertain whether American Roland would come through with an acceptable supply of lecithin. If the material was merely an approximation of the Shinitzky formula, would it be acceptable? Tom had taken the initiative for the project; he would bear any blame. Anything could happen at the last minute.

And something did happen.

Sonnabend had been satisfied with the laboratory report on a sample provided in advance by American Roland. Skornik declared that a further sample sent to Israel by air express did differ in appearance and odor from the Israeli product, but he found the material generally satisfactory and recommended that it be distributed. Sonnabend insisted, however, upon a further test of the shipment itself. Unfortunately, the truck did not arrive until late Thursday afternoon (April 23), the day before the distribution, too late for a laboratory test. Sonnabend would not authorize a distribution for the next day.

Two hundred people were expected to assemble at the Judson Memorial Church in the morning, some arriving from as far away as Texas.

Arnold Forster, for several decades chief counsel for the Anti-Defamation League of the B'nai Brith, had expressed concern that Praxis might attempt some legal action to block the distribution. He promised that in such an event he would defend the group pro bono. Early Friday morning (April 24), Tom called Forster. After a twenty-minute conversation, Arnold was not sure what Tom, sputtering with anxiety, wanted from him.

The night before, it appeared, Tom had attempted to contact Arnold Lippa, the president of Praxis, to ask him to test the Roland lecithin at the City University of New York so that Sonnabend would grant authorization for its distribution the next morning. Failing to reach Lippa, Tom called Praxis headquarters in Los Angeles. When a secretary at last realized that Tom was talking about a distribution of an AL721 analog to two hundred people, she connected him with James Jacobson, Jr., and he, in turn, instructed her to find Lippa.

The conversation began at 8 P.M. and lasted almost an hour.

The secretary was unable to reach Lippa.

At about 1 in the morning, Jacobson called Tom. Tom asked Jacobson to supply a quantity of AL721 for the next day's distribution. As the conversation continued with no resolution, Tom became increasingly impassioned. "All these months you could have made the substance available," he declared, "and didn't do so. Because of this negligence you may have contributed to the death of thousands of people. Please don't say that we are on the same side unless you intend to make the material available immediately to people who need it. You'll never be on the same side as the people who have died."

Jacobson was taken aback but made no promises. When Tom begged for help, Jacobson expressed sympathy but kept repeating, "There are things happening right now that I just can't talk about."

Tom declared that the PWA Health Group would go ahead with a press conference called for the next morning. Jacobson appealed to Tom not to announce that American Roland had no fear of the AL721 patent.

Tom refused.

The next morning, having given away his trump card—a threat to challenge the patent—Tom wanted clarification regarding the validity of the patent before the start of the press conference. Arnold put the group's lawyer in touch with one of New York's leading patent experts. This lawyer was of the opinion that since American Roland and other firms had been producing egg lecithin commercially long before the development of AL721 Praxis would not risk a confrontation on the issue.

Friday morning, April 25, with no AL721 authorized by Sonnabend ready for distribution, Michael Callen opened the press conference with a prepared statement—in effect, a PWA declaration of policy:

> We believe that any substance or intervention which has no or extremely low toxicity and has a rational theoretical possibility of doing some good ought to be available to People with AIDS and others who desire to obtain such interventions. . . . Why, you may ask, have People with AIDS been unable to obtain a food substance which may well save their lives? Why have some PWAs been forced to risk their lives boiling acetone to extract lecithin from egg yolks? . . . Why do PWAs themselves have to take time and energy from their own individual struggles for survival to do the job that others are supposed to be doing? . . . If egg lecithin turns out to benefit people with AIDS, then every day Praxis and the FDA and the NIH wait, more will needlessly die. . . .

He went on to say:

> I always assumed that good old corporate greed would speed up finding treatments for AIDS. By floating the merest whisper that we had found a company who would sell us an analog of AL721, we had $20,000 in orders within 24 hours. We have received desperate calls from Florida, Texas, California, Hawaii and Europe. . . . We hope not to be in this "business" long.

We hope that others—perhaps health food stores—will jump on the bandwagon and we can get out. Better yet, with your help, maybe we can shame the federal government into getting serious about testing egg yolk lecithin in the treatment and prevention of AIDS!

The press conference failed. "Not a peep in the papers," said Michael. "People seemed to feel that it was a non-story since delivery had not taken place." The group had to recontact everyone who had sent in a check for the material.

Two of the PWAs who had ordered the lipids died before the new distribution set for May 4.

6

CHAPTER

Who Will Supply AL721 to the PWAs?

The American Connection

Until the publicity about Michael May's "recovery," the AIDS community was unaware that AL721 had already been used with apparent success with an HIV-infected individual and that the development of the Israeli therapy was being frustrated by James Jacobson, Jr., the general licensee for the substance.

How was it possible that officials at Yeda, the commercial arm of the Weizmann Institute—men who over many years had been promoting products produced in Institute laboratories—should have exhibited such ignorance of the complications involved in establishing a pharmaceutical firm, developing production and distribution facilities and obtaining governmental authorization of a new pharmaceutical as to entrust these responsibilities to a 28-year-old man with no experience whatsoever in manufacturing, much less in pharmaceuticals?

As evidence of his involvement with "science," James A. Jacobson, Jr., known to friends and foes as "Jake," declared in his company's prospectus that in 1978, at the age of 26, he founded "FFGB" as "a non-profit foundation established to sponsor the educational processes and new research in the medical field." Questioned about the foundation, unlisted in any reference work, Linda Hunt, the public relations officer for Praxis, Jacobson's firm, replied, "I don't remember what the letters stand for, and I always forget to ask Jake."

Aside from inherited wealth (his grandfather gained a fortune from Sealy mattresses and his father from a leveraged buyout of Pocket Books), what qualifications had Jacobson to recommend him to obtain the Israeli license to manufacture and distribute AL721 throughout the world? A rumor, confirmed by Hunt, held that he was granted the license because his family had raised millions of dollars for the Weizmann Institute. Meir Shinitzky, however, flatly denied that Jacobson's family had made any such generous donation.

According to Bill Regelson of the Medical College of Virginia, David Samuel introduced Jake to David Heron, the graduate student whom Shinitzky and Samuel assigned to conduct AL721 experiments on brain membranes. Heron was dazzled by Jake's yuppie "ideals," and he shared Jake's interest in parapsychology. (George Krsek, one of Jacobson's initial consultants, reports that Jacobson was once incommunicado for several weeks, off with his wife on a spiritual retreat.) Heron was invited to a Jacobson country home that covers half a mountain at Ojai in northern California. Jacobson's wife was a medium and a disciple of Yuri Gellert, an Israeli who enjoyed a large following in parapsychology circles because of his supposed ability to bend spoons through mental concentration. At a seance, at Heron's request, Jacobson's wife asked Astronin, her contact with the Beyond, to explain the operating principle behind AL721. "Electricity," replied Astronin. "You see, Shinitzky," exclaimed Heron, "that's the way to go!"

In 1981, impressed by Heron's enthusiasm regarding the potential in AL721 for treating geriatric disorders as well as drug addiction and alcoholism, Jacobson applied for the license to manufacture and distribute the substance and offered to outbid any proposal from A. Natterman & Cie GmbH., a reputable German firm with which the Israelis were then negotiating. Just as the Israelis were about to sign a contract, the Germans noted that in the association they would be in violation of the Arab embargo. They proposed establishing a dummy company to serve as an intermediary. The Israelis broke off discussions.

Jacobson made promises—of a new research institute and of research funds. "The world is full of promises," commented Shinitzky belatedly. "Armand Hammer," the oil tycoon, he noted, "once promised five million dollars for cancer research. He got publicity in the newspapers, but the money never arrived."

In December 1981 the Israelis granted Jacobson a universal license for AL721.

On April 12, 1983, almost a year and a half later, Jacobson registered the Natural Pharmaceutical Corporation (NPC) in California "to further the research and development of AL and to act as the exclusive and worldwide licensee of AL." In September and December two subsidiary companies were formed: Matrix Research Laboratories, Inc., "to conduct and supervise the research and development"; and Active Lipid Development Partners, Ltd. (ALDP), "to perform certain research and development on AL."

NPC voted Jacobson over $300,000, a sum representing, plus interest, what he had advanced to the Israelis both for the license and for research projects. In April the company sold 900 shares of common stock to Jacobson for $9,000 in cash. In October the board of directors approved a stock split with an exchange of 100 shares for each share of common stock. Jacobson then sold 4,293 of his 90,000 shares to his uncle Leslie A. Jacobson for $2,147 and 2,576 shares to the principals of the company's legal counsel, Tilles & Webb, for $4,500. With these transactions, Jacobson recouped $6,647 of the $9,000 he had paid for his original 900 shares and retained possession of 83,131 shares.

◆ ◆ ◆

In 1982 Jacobson brought Heron to a scientific conference in Ventura, California. A flamboyant young man and a persuasive speaker, Heron impressed the assembled scientists with a model of the functioning of AL721 on membranes. When people addressed him as Dr. Heron, he did not correct them although he had not yet obtained his degree. Claude Baxter, a distinguished research scientist at the Veterans Administration Medical Center at Sepulveda, California, invited Heron to speak at his institution and then obtained an invitation for him to lecture at the University of California at Los Angeles.

Having read Shinitzky's reports on the effect of AL721 on the aging process, Bill Regelson sought out Heron for further information regarding possible collaboration with the Fund for Integrative Biomedical Research, a foundation promoting research in the biology of aging. At a dinner meeting, Regelson listened as Jacobson recounted grandiose promises he had made to Heron. Heron was to hold a leading post in the new institute Jacobson was going to establish at the Weizmann Institute and to carry on various research projects Jacobson was also going to fund.[1]

When Regelson offered the facilities and contacts of his foundation for promoting research on AL721, Jacobson was not receptive. He did agree to compensate Regelson for drafting an Investigational New Drug (IND) submission to FDA and promised to organize a fundraising dinner in Los Angeles for Regelson's foundation (never held).

On May 18, 1983 an IND drafted by Regelson was submitted to FDA for a clinical test of an oral formulation of AL721 in the therapeutic treatment of patients suffering from alcohol and methadone withdrawal.

Regelson put Jacobson in touch with Dr. Norman Applezweig, a consultant for pharmaceutical firms. When asked what abilities or experience Jacobson brought to his new venture, Applezweig retorted, "Absolutely nothing! I was hired as a consultant, but I had to take over the entire operation.

"I did not particularly like Jacobson," Applezweig added. "You could never get a straight answer from him. It was not that he was arrogant; he was evasive."

At Applezweig's suggestion, Jacobson obtained the services of Dr. George Krsek, the president of Houba, Inc. According to a Praxis company report of June 30, 1985, Krsek had had a long career with leading drug and pharmaceutical companies in "technical operations and policies, including research and development, clinical research, quality control, regulatory affairs, engineering and production." Krsek de-

---

[1] Jacobson kept none of his promises to Heron, who subsequently underwent a psychological crisis. He ceased pursuing his doctorate and dropped out of scientific life.

scribes his company as a "chemical and pharmaceutical firm where we specialize in nothing. We make up orders for particular items for other companies or institutions."

Like Applezweig, Krsek found Jake's ignorance impressive. "He didn't know shit from shinola," says Krsek. Jacobson wanted an analysis and then a sample of five kilos of AL721. He also asked Krsek to draft plans for the construction of a plant to produce AL721. Krsek gave an estimate of $1 million for the project. Jacobson, ever eager to cut corners, turned to a California contractor willing to do the work for a mere $150,000. Krsek discovered that the man knew nothing about manufacturing pharmaceuticals. Dissuaded from dealing with this man, Jacobson opened negotiations with a contractor in New Jersey equally ignorant of the field. The man called Krsek once for advice and never called back.

During 1983 and 1984, in consultation with Regelson and Applezweig, Jacobson sponsored a series of clinical tests with AL721. Ignoring the common practice of established pharmaceutical firms, Jacobson supplied the material but offered few or no research funds in subsidy. When he sent a small quantity of AL721 to Baxter at the VA Medical Center in Sepulveda, California for a research project, he said that for administrative reasons he would have to charge Baxter $20 for the material but would reimburse him for that amount forthwith. Baxter sent a check but never recovered the amount.

At Regelson's suggestion, Jacobson asked Bernard Bihari, director of the Kings County Addictive Disease Clinic at the Health Science Center in Brooklyn, New York, to draft a protocol for a clinical study of AL721 in withdrawal from drug addiction. Jacobson also approached research scientists at Wayne State University and at New York University to draft protocols for research in Alzheimer's disease. Subsequent Praxis reports make no mention of any follow-up on these initiatives.

According to Bihari, "Jacobson could have made a fortune if he had pursued the investigation of AL721 in the treatment of addicts and alcoholics."

For drafting a protocol for an FDA Phase I trial (a test for toxicity) Jacobson promised Bihari $5,000. The money was never paid, and Bihari heard no more from Jacobson about the protocol. "That was the pattern all along," Bihari declared, "calling and asking for something and then not calling back."

On a visit to Lederle Laboratories to seek collaboration with Jacobson's firm, Applezweig met Arnold S. Lippa. Lippa struck Applezweig as an energetic entrepreneur with a will and ability to make money, a man with the experience and decisiveness lacking in Jacobson. No monkish researcher, Lippa had broken with his Orthodox Jewish background. (His father had survived the Holocaust by escaping from a Nazi concentration camp.) Lippa drove an Alfa Romeo and was frequently caught in highway speed traps. Among friends and acquaintances, he had a reputation as an ace wheeler-dealer.

Having tested AL721 in his laboratory, Lippa was convinced of its potential and was eager to be associated with its development. On August 15, 1984 Lippa signed a five-year contract with Jacobson, and two weeks later, on August 28, the company was reorganized under the name Praxis Pharmaceuticals, Inc. As of January 1985,

Lippa was to become president and Jacobson, chairman of the board. Lippa was to receive a salary equal to Jacobson's of $75,000 per year with a ten percent increment each year thereafter. Meanwhile, for the remainder of 1984, both men obtained salaries from Matrix Laboratories, the firm's wholly owned subsidiary.

The Israelis were reassured by Lippa's association with the firm. Regelson called him a genius and an outstanding neurophysiologist with a tremendous drive, and Krsek, who had no warm personal feelings for Lippa, characterized him as an exceptional scientist. (Applezweig, who quickly developed an antipathy toward Lippa, thought Krsek's characterization exaggerated.) With Lippa's appointment, Regelson believed that the company was "finally on track."

◆ ◆ ◆

Financial matters were not neglected in the reorganization. For his holdings in NPC Jacobson obtained 3,315,084 shares in newly formed Praxis and 18,791 for his interests in ALDP, for a total of 3,333,875 shares. Jake's uncle Leslie A. Jacobson received 177,130 shares for his NPC interests; and members of the company's law firm received 106,204 shares for their NPC and 18,791 shares for their ALDP holdings. During the last six months of 1984 the new company repaid Jacobson $200,000 of monies he had previously advanced and agreed to pay a balance of $115,750 with accrued interest by June 1986.

In September 1984, in advance of a public stock offering of 767,050 shares projected for the following year, the directors of the new corporation authorized Jacobson to purchase 5,000 shares in the new company for $5,000. Lippa received an option to purchase 550,000 shares of company stock at $.01 per share in annual instalments of 110,000 shares commencing January 17, 1985, the date declared effective by the Securities and Exchange Commission for a public stock offering. In addition, he was granted a relocation loan of $100,000 with the expectation, however, that the company would grant him "from time to time bonuses in an amount sufficient to repay this obligation."

In January 1985 Lippa received 110,000 shares of common stock valued at $165,000 in exchange for his assignment of a letter of intent for a research and development contract with Receptor Technologies, Inc. (RTI), of which Lippa was a founder and a major shareholder. When RTI failed to complete a private placement to finance research and development expenditures, Praxis took "proprietary rights in and to the laboratory automation system and the other proposed RTI projects."

In February 1985 shares sold at $6 in a public offering (netting $3,683,599) were diluted in value by the hundreds of thousands of shares (620,000 in 1985 and an additional 59,000 in 1986) purchased or available for purchase through options at $.01. On the other hand, the shares purchased at minimal prices by officers and directors and "certain private investors" as well as those acquired at $.01 options were proportionately augmented in value in association with the shares sold in the public offering. By March 1987 the company's officers and directors and "certain private investors" owned 5,336,800 shares of the outstanding common stock purchased at an average of $.42 per share.

Such stock manipulations are common and legal in the United States. The impression for an outside observer, however, was that the corporation's board was devoting disproportionate time and energy to financial maneuverings.

First Experiment with HIV

In 1983 Regelson came upon an article by Mark Lyte, a former graduate student of Shinitzky's, in which Lyte contended that AL721 reduced the membrane rigidity of lymphocytes and thereby reduced immune deficiency in aging animals. Regelson called Bihari. "You have AIDS patients in your hospital," he said. "Why not ask Jacobson to test AL721 with them as well as with addicts?"

According to Bihari, "Bill Regelson was probably the first person who thought of using AL721 with AIDS. He told me, and I told Jacobson."

Jacobson ignored Bihari's suggestion.

Discovering that a friend he was treating for alcohol addiction was also suffering from AIDS Related Complex (ARC), Bihari decided to follow Regelson's suggestion without awaiting Jacobson's approval. He obtained a kilo of AL721 from Applezweig. According to Bihari, the patient "improved markedly until the material ran out."

Bihari reported his findings to Lippa, the new president and director of scientific research at Praxis. Lippa and Jacobson offered to supply Bihari with material to continue the treatment on condition that the patient allow them to publicize the case. When Bihari's friend, a man in a high government position, insisted upon confidentiality, Lippa and Jacobson refused to make more AL721 available for the treatment. (The man subsequently obtained the lipid variant from Tom Hannan's PWA Health Group.)

Lippa then asked Bihari to conduct a clinical trial of AL721 with AIDS.

Bihari expressed interest.

Lippa never followed up on his request.

Research for Better or for Worse

According to Krsek, "Lippa is an extremely good neurobiologist but not the man to run a company. I would send him copies of things," Krsek explained. "He would claim I had not sent them. 'Don't bother me if you don't know how to run your business,' he'd say. I would check with Federal Express and find the copies had been delivered. Then he'd say, 'Oh, I remember that.'" Like Applezweig and others, Krsek had financial problems with Jacobson and Lippa. "They would simply decide not to pay for a while."

Relations between Krsek and Lippa (who had already broken off relations with Applezweig) became particularly strained in 1986 when Lippa sent notices to researchers that fifty kilos of AL721 ordered for experiments did not meet specifications. Research work was halted until it was discovered that the error had been not in the manufacture but in a new method of assay introduced by Lippa. Krsek's materials *were* up to par.

Upon assuming office as president of the firm, Lippa tripled appropriations for research. In a January 1985 prospectus for a public stock offering filed with the Securities and Exchange Commission, the firm listed ten studies in progress. Of nine of the research scientists contacted in 1987 two declared that because of an agreement signed with Lippa they could not divulge the results of their studies without his acquiescence. One refused flatly to respond to any questions. Another, a member of Ethigen's Scientific Advisory Board, was suspicious and abrupt. His study, he said, had been abandoned after the advisory board voted in 1985 to focus all research on the treatment of AIDS. (In fact, eight other scientists did complete their studies, no one of which was related to AIDS.)

John Tew, a colleague of Regelson's at the Medical College of Virginia, recounted that the feed containing AL721 that he had been given resulted in an overdose of the lipids so that fat accumulated in the livers of the experimental animals. When he redid the experiment and sent a report to Lippa, he received no acknowledgment.

Israeli-born Robert Loria, also at the Medical College of Virginia, like Tew had problems with the AL721 animal feed Lippa provided. Krsek had formulated it for rats and not for the mice Loria used in his experiments. Like Tew, after a single association, Loria had no further communication with Lippa.

Loria subsequently, however, published data supporting Shinitzky's theory regarding the functioning of AL721. Loria demonstrated that animals fed a high-cholesterol diet become more susceptible to virus infection. A high-cholesterol diet, it appeared, is immuno-suppressive because of a change it effects in membrane fluidity. Loria published the results of a study in which he fed animals resistant to a certain virus a diet rich in cholesterol. After he increased the cholesterol to a certain level, the animals suffered 100 percent mortality from the virus. He then sought to find at what point the animals became susceptible to the virus, testing first after two and then after six and eight weeks, and so on. Next, reducing the cholesterol diet, he tested at what point the animals redeveloped resistance to the virus. According to Loria, significant scientific data existed to support the association between cholesterol and viral susceptibility.

John Rotrosen of the New York University School of Medicine obtained inconclusive results in a study of the effects of AL721 on alcohol withdrawal with mice. He was not able to confirm a similar Israeli study.

David Harrison of Jackson, Maine, had to wait so long for a supply of AL721 that the mice he assembled for the test aged too much—895 days instead of 500— for an effective experiment. He fed twenty-four mice for 225 days with material Lippa supplied and achieved a minimal result. He received no subsidy from Lippa.

Shinitzky considered of decisive importance the research conducted by Fulton Crews of the University of Florida Medical School at Gainesville. Crews and P. S. Sarin of the National Cancer Institute investigated AL721 as an immunal stimulant.

They confirmed experiments conducted at the Weizmann Institute and demonstrated further that AL721 acted as an antiviral agent. Upon their report of this discovery, Crews received an excited call from Lippa. "How is this possible?" Lippa exclaimed.

In the university library Crews found papers on arthritis and cancer published in the early 1970s by the researcher at the University of Virginia whose studies had inspired Shinitzky's investigations. Crews called Lippa and proposed the hypothesis of a lipid modification of viral receptors that inhibited the binding of the virus to cells and thus prevented infectivity. Lippa asked Crews to sign the Gallo letter about to be published in the *New England Journal of Medicine* in the fall of 1985, insisting that Gallo's in vitro study had developed out of Crews's investigation.

It was characteristic of the mode of operation at Praxis that Lippa did not inform Crews of Bihari's earlier successful AL721 experiment with a patient with HIV infection. Nor did Lippa inform the other members of the firm's Scientific Advisory Board that it was not Crews's findings alone that impelled Praxis, forced by its limited funds to concentrate its energies, to abandon AL721 investigations with drug addiction, alcoholism and geriatric disorders in favor of AIDS research.

"A Grave Social and Ethical Dilemma"

Early in the fall of 1984 Glen Mallory, a volunteer at the AIDS Medical Foundation (the forerunner to the American Foundation for AIDS Research), saw a notice in the *Wall Street Journal* of the organization of Praxis Pharmaceuticals as licensee for the manufacture and distribution of AL721. Mallory contacted the firm's president, Lippa. Lippa sent Mallory documents with information that would appear a year later in the Gallo letter to the *New England Journal of Medicine* along with reprints of papers by Shinitzky on the effects of the substance with geriatric patients with immune deficiency and on children with cystic fibrosis. Mallory relayed this material to Mathilde Krim and Joe Sonnabend.

Following upon the publication of the Gallo letter, Praxis began receiving requests for supplies of AL721. Testifying before the House Subcommittee of the Committee on Government Operations in July 1986, Lippa declared: "A day does not pass without inquiries from patients, parents, friends and doctors asking if there is a way for them to obtain AL721, knowing full well that it is still experimental." This situation, Lippa admitted, "poses a grave social and ethical dilemma for us."

Yet the extraordinary success of Burroughs Wellcome with AZT, the only AIDS drug then approved by FDA, apparently provided an irresistible temptation at Ethigen (the name newly adopted in place of Praxis). In May 1987 (the very month of the first PWA distribution in New York) the four members of the board of directors, informed that they would jeopardize their pursuit of FDA approval if they released AL721 as a food supplement, voted to reject a dual marketing approach. They refused to release the substance as a food supplement while simultaneously pursuing its authorization by the FDA as an ethical pharmaceutical.

Illusions at Ethigen

If the Ethigen directors were naive in their expectations of a sympathetic reception at FDA and a possible authorization of AL721 with the expedition FDA displayed with AZT, leaders of the AIDS community were not so unsophisticated. "The government," said Martin Delaney, "looks into a few narrowly defined products from the old-boy network and everything else gets the door slammed in its face."

To FDA and NIH officials Ethigen was no Burroughs Wellcome, no multinational giant. It was a new, untested company promoting a single health-food product, a pygmy operation with merely nine full-time employees (including its officers), without manufacturing facilities—a company organized by a millionaire with no experience or reputation. Furthermore, after maneuvering the publication in the prestigious *New England Journal of Medicine* of the Gallo letter urging investigation of AL721 as an AIDS therapy, Jacobson had been either unwilling or financially unable to promote a large multicenter clinical test that might have revealed, once and for all, the efficacy of his product.

Nor could the Ethigen officials mount a coordinated approach to FDA. A clash of personalities was unavoidable within this coterie of ambitious men of varying competence and experience compelled to assume diverse responsibilities in drawn-out, complex operations. Over the years Jacobson, adept at concealing his intentions, and the brash Lippa, separately or in concourse, antagonized numerous scientists, consultants and businessmen. A confrontation was inevitable between the two of them.

In August 1987, an SEC submission reported: "the Company . . . is modifying and/or transferring certain operational and scientific responsibilities from Dr. Lippa to Dr. Laskin and other members of management. . . . [t]here can be no assurance that Dr. Lippa will remain in the employ of the Company in any capacity during the full five year term of the agreement through January 17, 1990." Scientists and others associated with the enterprise, including the Israelis, as well, undoubtedly, as officials at NIH and FDA, had considered that Lippa's association with the firm rendered success of the venture more likely. Jacobson apparently no longer shared this opinion.

PWAs throughout the nation had no conception, of course, of the intrigues and financial maneuverings within the Israeli-licensed firm from which they awaited production and distribution of a therapy on which they laid great store for prolonging their lives.

AIDS Activists Take on
FDA and NIH

O n the ABC News "Nightline" television
program of July 27, 1987, at which Martin Delaney of Project Inform and FDA Commissioner Frank Young were appearing as guests, moderator Hodding Carter opened
with a challenge to the commissioner: "While no one yet claims a cure for AIDS,
there are several experimental drugs that prolong life, and all but one are caught in
a web of federal procedures that has kept them away from AIDS sufferers."

The program announcer intervened with a critical comment:

> In 1954, the federal government was quick to respond to the polio epidemic. A
> vaccine was approved and marketed after only four months of testing. 7,500
> people died of polio during the early 1950's. So far, AIDS has claimed 22,000
> lives. For someone dying of AIDS, even for someone in the preliminary stages of
> the disease . . . the wait for drugs can be agonizing and possibly fatal.

Young gave his standard response, pointing to the rapid approval accorded AZT as
an example of FDA expedition in bringing "breakthrough drugs to desperately ill
people. Right now," he declared, "there are no applications for pending approval for
actual completed studies."

Countering that there were "a dozen or more drugs that have sat around untested year after year," Delaney charged that the decisive problem was "that no one
is in charge, no one is leading this effort, no one is coordinating the pharmaceutical
companies with the National Institutes of Health."

To this astute and fundamental criticism Young could only reply that "going
too rapidly merely will lead to the same tragedies that were seen with HPA-23[1] and
Suramin, where a lot of people took a drug that was harmful."

---

[1] Developed at the Pasteur Institute, HPA-23 became famous when actor Rock Hudson flew to Paris in a
desperate and vain search for a cure for AIDS.

Delaney was not unsophisticated about Suramin, a drug used for some fifty years as a treatment for various tropical diseases. Two years earlier Delaney's lover, a PWA who had been progressing well on Ribavirin, was enrolled by doctors at San Francisco General Hospital in a Suramin study. After most of the sixteen participants were taken off the drug in about three months because of severe side effects, the doctors kept Delaney's lover on the treatment. As months passed, he became increasingly ill, and the day before Thanksgiving, Delaney carried him semicomatose to the hospital.

"Do something," Delaney demanded. "Look at him!"

"You guys are complainers," said the doctors. "It's nothing but a case of the flu."

Delaney raised a furor.

In the hospital records, a doctor found a test taken more than a month earlier showing almost complete adrenal failure.

Of the initial sixteen patients, only three or four survived the trial.

A year later in France, Delaney encountered two PWAs from Alabama who had been taking Suramin for more than a year under the supervision of a French physician. The French, it appeared, had discovered the drug to be effective in a lower dosage and prescribed biweekly instead of weekly.

In a conversation with Bill Regelson, Samuel Broder of the National Cancer Institute admitted that Suramin was not dangerous in itself. "You have to know how to use it," said Broder.

"It's certainly less toxic than AZT," commented Regelson, "but AZT is Broder's drug. If in this crisis NCI is involved with self-interest, who's going to find the alternative therapies?"

In the July 15, 1988 issue of *AIDS Treatment News*, John James summarized an article on Suramin by a Charles Lineberger appearing in the July/August issue of *San Francisco: The Magazine* in which the author charged that if the National Institutes of Health had issued a warning that symptoms of adrenal insufficiency, a possible side effect of Suramin, can mimic AIDS symptoms, the physicians running the trials would have tested regularly for adrenal damage and avoided or reduced the drug's dangerous side effects. Nevertheless, FDA repeatedly used the Suramin clinical test disaster as an excuse for delaying the release of other drugs.

Regelson recounts frustrating experiences with bureaucratic rigidity in regard to cancer drugs. On one occasion, after the condition of a patient he had sent by air ambulance to Mount Sinai Hospital in New York for treatment with an experimental cancer therapy stabilized, Regelson asked that the treatment be continued. The physician expressed regret. Having found out that he had accepted eighty-four patients for treatment instead of the sixty stipulated in the protocol, NCI had suspended his license for the treatment.

In an interview appearing in the *New York Times* on February 8, 1988, Dr. Robert K. Oldham, scientific director of Biotherapeutics, Inc. of Franklin, Tennessee, who had spent some eight or nine years on the staff of the National Cancer Institute and from 1980 to 1984 had served as organizer and director of the Institute's biological response modifiers program, described NCI as "a real closed shop in terms of thought processes," where staff have worked all their lives, spending little time at universities or in the private sector. "They're very focused on what they do at the NIH or NCI, and I think they have a little trouble seeing the forest for the trees. They're very suspicious that things done outside have somehow got a prurient kind of goal and that they really are the white knights."

Richard Dunne, executive director of the Gay Men's Health Crisis, summed up the view of the AIDS community regarding FDA and NIH: "Researchers don't seem to understand at a feeling level the predicament of a dying person who hears of something promising. Patients ought to be offered virtually anything that holds any promise of being effective. Human beings have a right to make their own decisions."

On Opposite Sides of the Table

In the spring of 1987, seeking to confront officials of NIH and FDA with the complaints and concerns in the AIDS community, Nathan Kolodner, president of the board of the Gay Men's Health Crisis, invited Larry Kramer, one of the founders both of the GMHC and of ACT UP, and two PWAs (Michael Callen, a founder of the PWA Coalition and of the PWA Health Group, and Dr. Barry Gingell, director of medical information for the GMHC) to join him in seeking a meeting with Dr. Anthony Fauci, the director of the National Institute for Allergies and Infectious Diseases (NIAID).

Having participated two weeks earlier in the PWA Health Group mass distribution of AL721, Callen had particular questions for Fauci about the lethargic promotion of new AIDS therapies. Gingell had a private as well as a professional interest in the forthcoming discussion. As a physician he had treated some twenty AIDS patients and three times that number with ARC. In 1984, at 30 years of age, he himself had fallen ill, suffering bouts of herpes and PCP. He made repeated trips to Mexico to obtain supplies of Ribavirin. Subsequently he had begun treatment with AZT and then with AL721.

A month earlier while researching an investigative story for *Newsday* on "who in Washington was in charge of the 'AIDS show,'" Larry Kramer had asked Gary Bauer, 41, an adviser to President Reagan on domestic issues, why there was no coordinated campaign against the epidemic directed by an individual with clearly defined authority. Bauer replied, "Our belief is that the president is that already, the AIDS czar." Bauer, Kramer discovered, did not know the precise initials of AZT, the single drug authorized by FDA for AIDS treatment, calling the drug instead "ACT." He had never heard of AL721.

Kramer was not granted an interview with Otis R. Bowen, the Secretary of Health and Human Services, but he did speak with Assistant Secretary of Health Robert E. Windom. Of Windom, who had been chairman of the Committee to Reelect Reagan and Bush in Florida, Georgia and Alabama, a congressional aide declared, "If his IQ were any lower, you'd have to water him"; and one of Windom's colleagues said of him, "a warm, affable, back-slapping fellow, but he's out of his league." When Kramer asked Windom why more drugs were not being tested, Windom replied, "We have a task force for that." Questioned why money appropriated for AIDS treatment and research was not being spent, Windom answered, "We have a committee for that." Regarding AL721 Windom said, "I'm not familiar with the details on that."

A Reagan aide told Kramer: "God help us with the AIDS epidemic because the U.S. government won't. Washington is not interested in AIDS."

Fauci, in charge of AIDS research for NIH, avoided confrontations. On April 1, on the Phil Donahue television show, Kramer and Martin Delaney, co-director of the San Francisco Project Inform, issued a challenge to Fauci (who had been invited to participate on the show but had failed to appear) to meet them publicly to debate issues relating to the testing and authorization of drugs.

Fauci was to appear with Delaney on the ABC "Nightline" show on July 27, but five minutes before the program started, Commissioner Frank Young of FDA appeared instead. Fauci, Young explained, was busy and at the last minute had asked him to fill in.

When appearing alone on television, said Kramer, "Fauci takes control, he has an answer for everything, he's very opinionated, he smiles at you, you can't budge him." "Fauci gets off easy," agrees Delaney. "He's attractive, and he's a high-level official. All the reporters go gaga. They take his word as final. We would like to put him on the spot and challenge what he says before the public."

Upon arriving for their meeting with Fauci at the Bethesda headquarters of the National Institutes of Health, Kolodner, Kramer, Callen and Gingell were gratified to discover that Fauci had assembled eleven colleagues from NIH and FDA.

For two hours the two groups faced each other across a conference table.

The general response to the gay activists' questions regarding the delay in promoting new AIDS therapies was that because there was substantive evidence that AZT was effective against the AIDS virus, NIH had set its focus and priority on that drug. More testing was required with AZT alone and in combination with other drugs. Other drugs would have to wait their turn.

When challenged as to why with the generous funding for AIDS research so little had been accomplished, Fauci and his colleagues insisted they were hampered by a shortage of staff and by the refusal of the Office of Management and Budget (OMB) to grant them more office space. (Kramer later observed that while complaining that his institute is shorthanded, "Fauci and his colleagues fly about the country granting interviews to press and television, lecturing and appearing on talk shows. You wonder who's minding the store. If you want an appointment, you don't call their secretaries, you call their press officers, who book their talks and interviews . . . like movie stars."[2])

---

[2] In response to a request for a list of Fauci's speaking engagements during 1987 Elaine Baldwin, a public relations person at NIAID, "stonewalled," repeatedly failing to return telephone calls. Finally she declared:

Callen suggested to the assembled officials that they line up promising drugs according to both their antiviral efficacy and their toxicity. "As a person with AIDS," he said, "I would prefer that you begin down the line with drugs with low toxicity and some or low anti-viral activity rather than with blow torches that are also very toxic." (Callen was alluding to AZT, effective with only about 40 percent of AIDS patients.)

"In a disease that's a number one health priority," noted Gingell, "for which so much money has been expended, there should be enough manpower and facilities to look at a drug [AL721] that appears promising before two years elapse after a recommendation from Gallo and the others."

When Callen pressed Fauci further on AL721, Fauci exploded. "See," he exclaimed, "that's a perfect example. Our committee considered it. There's no evidence that it works whatsoever. Because of all the brouhaha that you've created [the publicity regarding the PWA Health Group's distribution of an AL721 analog], we looked at it again."

"What about the Weizmann Institute studies, what about Gallo's letter?" demanded Callen. "Are you saying that Gallo is publishing shit?"

"The Weizmann data is nonsense, useless," replied Fauci. As for the Gallo letter, he declared: "If I take a tube of blood from a person with AIDS and I put oregano in it, it will probably kill the virus. If I had to sit up and take notice of every substance in a test tube. . . ." Nevertheless, Fauci added, "We'll start animal toxicity trials because there is no data on AL721."

Having endured the ravages of AIDS for five years, Callen would not submit to Fauci's patronizing. "One of the foremost AIDS scientists publishes something almost two years ago saying that AL721 is a promising candidate as a treatment for AIDS," he exclaimed, "and I am now told that a Phase I toxicity study is only now beginning, and *that* because I have made a stink. . . ."

When Gingell commented that egg lecithin was not a toxic substance, Maureen W. Myers, chief of the AIDS Treatment Branch of NIAID, responded that the toxicity of AL721 had not been tested.

Kramer also was angered by Fauci's announcement of a toxicity trial for AL721. In March in an Op Ed piece in the *New York Times* Kramer had attacked FDA for its inertia in promoting promising AIDS therapies. The piece was followed by an ACT UP demonstration on Wall Street. When, a week later, Fauci announced he was going to release AL721 and another drug for clinical testing, Kramer called to congratulate Fauci. "How many people are you going to put on AL721?" he asked. "Will you have a hundred in the test?"

"We do not think that such information would put in perspective Dr. Fauci's major activities." Reminded that NIAID was not a private agency but a public institution with an obligation to make such information available, Ms. Baldwin promised to convey this message to her superior and to call back. She never called. A subsequent attempt to obtain the information under the Freedom of Information Act proved equally futile.

"We have to put it in Phase I, and so we're going to test it only on six," replied Fauci.

"It's already been in Phase I," Kramer declared.

"What do you mean?" asked Fauci.

"Michael Lange conducted it here in New York during the summer of 1986," said Kramer, "and it's now continuing in a second stage."

There was a long pause.

"I'm not familiar with that study," said Fauci.

"That study," Kramer said, "has been on your desk for three months."

"Well, I'll have to check into it," Fauci replied.

Now, two months later, Kramer discovered that Fauci was considering initiating a mere animal toxicity test![3]

To Fauci's insistence that a clinical test for AL721 had been delayed because Ethigen had failed to provide an acceptable placebo for a double-blind test, the AIDS activists responded: "Why would anyone be willing to take a placebo when they can make or buy the material on their own?"

Noting that pneumocystis carinii pneumonia (PCP) was the major cause of death for PWAs, Callen urged Fauci to issue interim prophylaxis recommendations in keeping with the experience of many New York clinicians. Fauci replied that without "hard data" he could not take the issue of prophylaxis seriously. "There isn't a doctor in New York," retorted Gingell, "who does not prescribe prophylaxis now." Indeed, Gingell pointed out, bactrim represented a case where an overwhelming body of anecdotal evidence could substitute for a double-blind study.

Fauci and one of his associates appealed to Callen "to go back to your [New York PWA] community and beg them to stop taking all these substances so that we [Fauci and his associates] can get clean data [in future clinical trials]." PWAs were even to go off prophylaxis!

"This was the only point during the meeting when I got really furious," recalled Callen. "Not only will I not do this," he declared, "but I am telling people to lie to get into your protocols, and it is your responsibility as scientists to design protocols broad enough to deal with all the variables.

"If you had this disease," cried Callen, "would you go off prophylaxis, would you take AL721?"

"I probably would," replied Fauci, "but that doesn't make it right."

(A month later in a discussion with another delegation of New York activists,

---

[3] Upon being told of the statement that the toxicity of AL721 had never been tested and that Fauci was planning to hold a toxicity clinical test, Fulton Crews of the University of Florida Medical School at Gainesville, one of the signers of the Gallo letter published in the *New England Journal of Medicine*, expressed astonishment. Bill Regelson of the Medical College of Virginia responded similarly. "Isn't that ironic," he declared, "especially when their AZT is as toxic as all hell?" Searching in his files, Regelson found the docket numbers of toxicity tests of egg lecithin conducted in 1979 by a committee set up by FDA under contract with the Federation of American Scientists, tests that demonstrated that the substance was harmless except when ingested in massive doses.

Fauci declared that they were fools to advocate the use of aerosolized pentamedine, a drug widely prescribed by New York physicians as a prophylaxis against PCP, inasmuch as no study had shown its value and doctors prescribing it might be putting their patients at risk. Five months later, when the *New England Journal of Medicine* published an editorial recommending pneumocystis prophylaxis as standard therapy for PWAs, Fauci, without apology or admission of error, made a complete and belated reversal in his stance.)

Gingell left the two-hour meeting in Bethesda with the impression that Fauci and his colleagues were isolated from the AIDS reality. "They design protocols mechanically," he said, "not around people or with the goal of saving lives."

As far as the delegation was concerned, remarked Kramer, "the meeting proved to be a total waste of time."[4]

An ATEU Test of AL721

Fearing ridicule for performing a superfluous toxicity test with an egg lecithin variant, in June 1987 FDA approved not a six-patient toxicity trial but a short-term dosage-ranging AIDS Treatment Evaluation Unit (ATEU) study involving sixty PGL (lymphodenopathy) and ARC patients. Some weeks later NIH announced an expansion of the test into a multicenter study to commence in September.

In mid-October, however, NIH imposed a hold on the tests because Ethigen had delivered a supply of AL721 from sources (Abbott Laboratories and Pfizer) other than the manufacturer (Houba) listed in the company's original clinical trials proposal. On November 12, unaware of this development, Tom Hannan, director of the Community Research Initiative in New York, called Dr. Donna Mildvan at Mt. Sinai Hospital to check on the progress of the AL721 study. Dr. Mildvan reported that she was still awaiting a supply of the substance.

From Dale Sprigg of NIAID Hannan learned that the supply of AL721 received from Abbott Laboratories was contaminated. A subsequent, satisfactory shipment had arrived for distribution to laboratories engaged in the ATEU study. "What kind of firm is this that handles its affairs so sloppily?" exclaimed Sprigg. "First Ethigen puts down Houba as its supplier, then they change to Abbott and then to Pfizer. Their first shipment is contaminated!"

When Hannan noted that the New York hospitals assigned to hold clinical tests had not received supplies, Sprigg replied that it was necessary for the researchers to submit a formal request for an allocation along with a list of patient participants. Hannan immediately called Dr. Henry Sack, the chief researcher at Beth Israel, and discovered that Sack was not aware of this regulation. He might have waited indefinitely for the AL721 if Hannan had not given him this information!

---

[4] The account of this meeting along with comments by various distinguished scientists on the matters discussed was submitted to Fauci for comment and correction. Fauci and his colleagues ignored the communication.

To replace the Abbott product, Jacobson had been compelled to ask Krsek (despite their bad personal relations) to ship 320 kilos of AL721 stored in Houba refrigerators since early in the year. Although Ethigen had a long-outstanding bill of $7,000 with Houba, Krsek complied with the request. "What was worse," Krsek admitted months later, berating himself for his naiveté, "they said that they had to have the material on Friday. I said that a rush order would cost another $1,000. They said, 'We authorize the extra cost, ship it.' So I shipped it, and they still haven't paid."

It would seem, however, that regardless of the results of these tests, AL721 could not hope for the enthusiastic promotion accorded AZT. At a November meeting of Americans for a Sound AIDS Policy, pressed by Bill Bahlman of the Lavender Hill Mob for an explanation of the failure to expedite the authorization of AL721, Robert C. Gallo of the National Cancer Institute responded testily: "I'll have you know that it was my paper on AL721 that brought it to the scientific community. There's very little usefulness in it."

Finally, in December, dosage-ranging studies began at Beth Israel and Memorial Sloan-Kettering in New York and at the University of Minnesota Health Science Center. Two months later, commenting on an interview with Fauci, the *New York Times* declared regarding the initiation of testing with AL721 that little could be expected from these trials inasmuch as "few if any officials expect the substance to prove effective, but they contend that a trial is needed because so many people are using it."

Speed-Up at FDA?

In a telephone conversation with Delaney on October 13, 1987 Boyden Gray, legal counsel to George Bush (whose campaign for nomination as a presidential candidate was then under way), expressed the vice president's frustration at FDA Commissioner Young's "sabotage" of new regulations governing the emergency release of experimental drugs, regulations first promoted by the vice president four years earlier. Bush, Gray said, was going to call for a Senate hearing on Young's half-hearted implementation of the new procedures.

From testimony of numerous witnesses at hearings conducted by the House Human Resources and Intergovernmental Relations Subcommittee on April 29, 1987 it was clear that FDA was being dragged along kicking and screaming by the Office of Management and Budget (OMB), a White House agency. A regulation drafted by the OMB prescribed that "FDA shall approve, for conditions that are life threatening and for which there is no satisfactory alternative drug or other therapy available, an application from a sponsor for treatment use of a drug that is under investigation in an approved IND [investigational new drug] study." Of the hearings on the new regulations, a Heritage Foundation study published precisely a year later, "Red Tape for the Dying: The Food & Drug Administration and AIDS," commented: "A well-orchestrated congressional hearing raised the specter of terminally ill patients being fleeced by unscrupulous drug companies—apparently this outweighed the reality of such individuals spending their last days ensnarled in red tape or left to the mercy of foreign or black market drug suppliers."

In the October 1987 issue of its publication "Perspective," Project Inform evaluated the amended regulation as follows:

> Young has said a treatment IND [as the new regulation was called] will only be considered when a drug has been proven effective in Phase II trials. . . . Many Phase II trials last longer than the average life expectancy of many PWAs. . . . The policy talks about *"the preponderance of scientific evidence, taken as a whole"* as the basis for determining efficacy. In practice, this has come to mean "whenever the Commissioner says so." . . . When the Commissioner disagrees with researchers, as is the case for at least one AIDS drug right now [Ribavirin], the Commissioner simply wins.

By the end of 1987 none of four drugs submitted for approval under the new regulation had been approved. Not a single person with AIDS had experienced any benefit from the "new" regulations.

National Gay Rights Advocates et al. vs. Department of HHS et al.

On a picket line outside the White House—one of the protest actions during the June 1987 International Conference on AIDS—Leonard Graff, the legal director for the National Gay Rights Advocates (NGRA), and Jean O'Leary, the organization's executive director, came up with the idea of a class action suit against agencies of the Department of Health and Human Services (HHS) on the charge of negligence in the testing and authorization of AIDS therapies.

Graff, 37, a gay activist for more than fifteen years, had agitated in Lansing, Michigan, for a municipal equal rights ordinance. Subsequently, as the first openly gay attorney in Washington, he engaged in pro bono work in defense of gay clients, and in 1982 he was appointed legal director for NGRA. After the White House picketing, Graff represented the sixty-four demonstrators who were arrested.

The NGRA litigation committee obtained the services of Forrest A. Hainline III, a member of a distinguished Washington law firm, and on June 24, a mere three weeks after the conclusion of the Washington international AIDS conference, Hainline filed a class action suit in the Federal District Court of the District of Columbia with a complaint against "defendants . . . Otis R. Bowen, M.D., in his official capacity as Secretary of HHS . . . Frank E. Young, M.D., in his official capacity as Commissioner of FDA . . . and James B. Wyngaarden, M.D., in his official capacity as Director [of the NIH]."

After citing Centers for Disease Control statistics on the rapid expansion of the AIDS epidemic, the plaintiffs noted: "In 1986 Congress appropriated $100 million to NIH to enable all AIDS patients to obtain treatment with experimental drugs. NIH has not expended these funds as Congress intended." The NGRA complaint charged also that "NIH concentrated its research into NIH-sponsored drugs or into drugs developed by companies with which NIH or its researchers had developed special relationships. . . . At the same time, NIH ignored or seriously delayed consideration and testing of promising drugs, even though those drugs were safer than those it chose to advance. . . ."

At the National Academy of Sciences conference on AIDS on September 1, 1987 Barry Gingell offered a summary criticism of the ATEU program, calling it a "dismal failure." He noted that with an enrollment of 1,200, the $47 million allocation represented a cost of $40,000 per patient in the trials. Ninety percent of the patients in NIH-sponsored trials were receiving AZT despite the evidence that up to 50 percent of patients cannot tolerate the drug and that at least seven other drugs on hand were deserving of study. "NIH," he concluded, "has put all its research eggs in one basket."[5]

As a result of what it characterized as "improper action and inaction by NIH and FDA," the NGRA complaint charged that "infected patients must take matters into their own hands, and either concoct home remedies, travel to foreign countries, or purchase unregulated drugs on the black market. In effect, NIH compels law-abiding citizens to become criminals in a desperate effort to save their own lives." The plaintiffs sought, among other actions, "an injunction requiring the defendants "to adopt, publish, and implement appropriate rules and regulations to ensure the effective operation of NIH with respect to its AIDS research mission, including public disclosure of the process for choosing drugs for testing, the reasons for drug selection, and the safety and effectiveness of drugs tested . . . [and] publicly to account for expenditure of funds appropriated by Congress for AIDS research and testing. . . ."

The NGRA suit represented a complement to, and a culmination of, protest actions by groups like the Lavender Hill Mob, ACT UP, and the San Francisco Mobilization Against AIDS as well as self-empowerment initiatives by the New York Persons with AIDS Coalition and similar groups throughout the nation. The class action suit exemplified and further impelled a change in atmosphere within the gay community and in its relations with the federal government.

◆ ◆ ◆

Although Hainline, the chief counsel in the NGRA case, and his associate Sherrie K. Kennedy were barred by court order from obtaining documents under the Freedom of Information Act pending a hearing on the defendants' motion for dismissal, they

---

[5] In March 1987 David Shuloff of Washington University in St. Louis applied for a grant for a research study of various drugs in combination. On October 1, receiving notice of an NIH grant of $4.5 million, Shuloff gave assignments to his staff. Two weeks later, however, he was informed that he could use the funding only for existing NIH protocols. In effect, he could duplicate trials already in progress, on AZT or derivatives of AZT. If he insisted upon pursuing the study in his application, previously approved, he would either lose his funding or mark time pending a reconsideration of his proposal at the next NIH meeting on ATEUs. Shuloff's was not a unique experience.

arrived at fundamental insights regarding the complaint. "A lot that is going on here is not peculiar to AIDS," declared Hainline during an interview in September 1987. "I am at present representing a company that makes a device that is in almost every doctor's office in Germany, Switzerland and France. Eventually it will be accepted here." FDA caution, he admitted, was desirable generally, but "when you have a group of people who have no hope, where you have a problem which, if not solved, will bring a disaster for society, more flexibility is required."

Hainline was struck by the insularity in federal health agencies, as exemplified in the fight between NIH scientists and scientists of the Pasteur Institute in Paris over who discovered HIV. "They are like a bunch of kids saying, 'This is my toy.' Such bickering is not only unseemly, but it supports my theory that these doctors are putting their own reputations and interests ahead of the development of cures or solutions to the AIDS disease. This is a world, not a United States, problem. Everything we learn here helps people everywhere. Everything learned elsewhere helps people here."

In defense of what appears to many as rigidity in its procedures, Hainline said, FDA points to its timely rejection of thalidomide, a drug that caused hundreds of cases of deformity among newborn infants in Europe. (Claude Baxter of the VA Medical Center in Sepulveda asserts that thalidomide was not approved in the United States only because FDA procrastinated in testing the drug until the dangers had become apparent overseas.) The individual infected with HIV, Hainline insisted, is not like a thalidomide victim, an infant with a chance of a normal life though with a possible deformity. The individual who has progressed to ARC or AIDS is told, "You will live anywhere from six months to two years. You are basically a walking dead man. A leper. Here's a bell. Let everyone know you're coming.

"Every time you test [a therapy] and fail, you have a chance of learning something. Researchers can give these people [infected with HIV] a chance to satisfy the most fundamental of all human needs—to be generous in spirit. We'll learn from this test and maybe five years from now because of you, someone else will live. . . .

"In Genesis," Hainline declared, "we are told that man is created in God's image. I think that's a call, an invitation. We all have the chance, opportunity and responsibility, a chance for care and hope."

CHAPTER 8

The PWAs Take Over

The Praxis/Ethigen decision to delay the production and distribution of AL721 until FDA authorized it as an AIDS therapy meant, in effect, that the AIDS community could not anticipate a supply from the firm for at least four or five years.

PWAs would not submit to procrastination with a therapy they believed offered hope of prolonging their lives. Indeed, *a major significance of the AL721 struggle lay in the impetus it provided to the organization of PWA distribution groups throughout the country.* The PWA Health Group in New York led the way.

For the $20,000 worth of lipids for the PWA Health Group's May 4, 1987 distribution, unusual preparations were required. A security officer of the Gay Community Center was hired, and the Gay [Police] Officers Action League agreed to have members look in at the Greenwich Village church where the distribution was to be held.

Following a second press conference, a few reports appeared in the media. A *Newsday* reporter quoted a spokesman at the Food and Drug Administration as saying that what the PWA Health Group was doing was probably illegal but that FDA was going to put its efforts into speeding up the processing of drugs rather than into pursuing punitive action against individuals who, the spokesman implied, were profiteering on the crisis.

On May 5 Hector Munoz was interviewed on a Spanish-language television channel. The telephone number of the PWA Coalition was flashed briefly on the screen as well as Hector's private number. Hector received about ten calls.

On May 10 under the heading "AIDS: Plague of the 80's," the *New York Daily News* carried a description of Jim Perez and Suzanne Phillips making the egg lecithin variant in Jim's apartment. The correspondent wrote:

Scoffing at sceptics, cancer-stricken James Perez has turned his dark, little fifth-floor flat into a "guerrilla lab" on the upper East Side. . . . Perez, 34, operates one of a growing number of clandestine labs nation-wide to make substances that the government has yet to approve and companies haven't even begun to manufacture. . . .

Dr. Anthony Fauci and Dr. Robert Gallo of the National Institutes of Health separately have acknowledged that egg-yolk lecithin, whether drug or food, is worth researching further. But people like Jim Perez and Sue, both of whom have lost friends to AIDS, do not have time to wait. Seated before 10 dozen eggs and two gallons of acetone, Sue declares while separating whites from yolks, "We're not talking about drugs, we're talking about food. It's eggs, for God's sake. . . . People like Jim are alive today because of what he and people who love him are doing." . . . [They will make] this day's product at a cost of about $35. Into the yolks she pours a gallon of flammable acetone, stirring constantly. . . . The solution, soon looking like egg-drop soup, is poured into a pillow case placed inside the wringer of the kind of pail used in mopping floors. The liquid is extracted, the solids are put through another acetone bath. This time the solids are thrown out and the liquid is saved.

The material is placed in the freezer overnight, the reporter continued. Then, "in the final step, the solution will be placed into a pump to extract all the acetone."

While the reporter was at the apartment, Ed, one of the Americans who had gone to Israel for treatment with AL721, arrived to pick up his dose, "for which he will not be charged, though he will buy yolks in bulk for his suppliers." "Taking this stuff is not foolhardy or desperate," the reporter quoted Ed as saying. "Anyone with a terminal illness should break all the rules. Rules do not apply when you don't have much time left."

Two days later, on May 12, 1987, the weekly *Voice* carried a story both on the May 4 distribution and on the newly formed Community Research Initiative. The reporter quoted Mathilde Krim as saying, "It's a great pity that AL721 is not studied on a wide scale." "Why shouldn't AL721 be made immediately available for every-one?" asked Joe Sonnabend. Michael Lange of St. Luke's/Roosevelt Hospital declared: "Since we've known about this for over two years, one can say: Why hasn't this been tried? What right do we have to withhold something that is harmless?"

The reporter attempted to question someone at Praxis/Ethigen as to its failure to market the substance. "Two officers of Praxis," he asserted, "refused comment and referred the inquiry to Praxis chairman James Jacobson. Linda Hunt, who handles public relations for the firm, said Jacobson was out of town."

◆ ◆ ◆

Reports of favorable results from the first egg lecithin distribution began arriving at the PWA Health Group office. A Hispanic woman tugged at Michael Callen's arm and said, "You saved my nephew's life. It works. You must know that. You must do everything to make this available."

Six weeks after Suzanne brought an initial batch of homemade lipids to the friend whose imminent death she was expecting at the time of the Michael May meeting, her friend's mother called. She was crying. Her son was out of bed! He was walking around the apartment! Without the assistance of a walker! He had gained thirteen pounds, and his psoriasis had cleared up. "I ran out to his house," Suzanne recounted, "with a bottle of champagne, and we celebrated."

Ron Monroe (the man who at the February 24 meeting had offered a copy of the AL721 patent to Suzanne) and his lover had constructed a lipid laboratory in their kitchen. By mid-August Ron's T4 cell count had quadrupled—an extraordinary improvement—and his T8 (suppressor) cells had decreased. He had not been sick in eight months, and his prime worry was the weight he was gaining.

Ron Monroe died in February 1990.

The most impressive transformation through the egg lecithin was described in the July 20 issue of the *New York Native*. One day late in May a PWA got out of bed, dressed, walked downstairs to the kitchen, and asked his lover: "Hey, aren't we supposed to be going somewhere? Aren't we going to California?" His lover looked at him with astonishment. These were the first sentences he had spoken in a month.

Upon the appearance of Kaposi's sarcoma lesions on the man's leg, his lover made four separate trips to Mexico for supplies of Ribavirin. Wracked by opportunistic infections, he lost weight, motor control and, most dismaying, his mind as well. He was unable to speak, to understand or to remember anything. By the time his lover obtained egg lecithin at the May 4 distribution, he was semicomatose. The lover force-fed him egg lecithin mixed with orange juice, squirting it into his mouth with a syringe. Sometimes the operation took hours. Within a month he was out of bed and able to remember some details from the past. By mid-July he was optimistic about the future. "I'm still a little spacy," he told the *Native* reporter, "but I *was* dying. My doctor says my recovery is miraculous, and now he is recommending the egg lecithin to other patients with AIDS."[1]

In mid-June the PWA Health Group held a second distribution of egg lecithin, this time to 900 people. On one of the worst days of an extraordinarily virulent heat wave, $100,000 worth of materials were sitting outside the Judson Memorial Church in a refrigeration truck. The security guard slept in the cab overnight.

On August 7 Hector Munoz finished the batch from the May 4 distribution. "It took me about two weeks," he said, "to pull myself together to mix the egg lecithin. I kept thinking of the bother of mixing and pouring the liquid into trays." The brother

---

[1] The "recovery" did not last. Within some weeks after the report in the *Native*, the man died. It was possible that he was too far gone for the effect to continue. It was also likely, as proponents of AL721 were beginning to suspect, that the lecithin should have been complemented with yet another drug for the best effect.

of a PWA friend of Hector's paid for a second batch. "He is just a boy who has a regular job and doesn't make much money," declared Hector. "He said, 'You're going to have it,' and he bought it for me."

Hector could not tell whether the lecithin had brought any improvement in his condition, "but many people," he said, "have noticed a change, people who haven't seen me for a long time. I'm strong, I'm not out of breath, I'm not tired. I don't suffer from sweating or from fevers."

Hector was receiving calls constantly from Hispanics inquiring about the AL721 analog. "Most of those who call are in the panic stage," said Hector, "suffering the first shock after diagnosis. There's little done for the Spanish-speaking people. They are badly organized. I don't have the strength to do the organizing myself." Nevertheless, city officials were arranging for Hector to address community groups. He had recently talked to some fifty women on the East Side of Manhattan. Hector spoke about sex frankly, and they, in turn, were very open in their questions. (Frankness about sexuality is rare among Hispanics.) At the end of his talk, Hector told the women that he had AIDS. "It was a very emotional moment," he said. "Many of them came and embraced me and cried and offered to help me."

Hector Munoz died on November 4, 1988.

Not all those who took the AL721 analog enjoyed such an extension of life. After undergoing surgery on internal Kaposi's sarcoma lesions, Jim Perez went home to Texas to spend some weeks with his family before reporting for another operation to remove a further lesion in his intestines. His internal lesions kept spreading, and he had increasing difficulty holding down food and medicine. One night in a dream he resolved the swallowing problem. He would take the lecithin in gelatine. The expedient worked.

Suzanne Phillips was to fly to Texas to bring Jim back to New York for his intestinal operation. She reported that Jim seemed semidelirious on the telephone. With an air ticket purchased for her by Ron Monroe and his lover and with a batch of an AL721 analog donated by the PWA Health Group and another batch made by Jim's friend Kevin Imbusch, Suzanne arrived at Jim's Texas town. He was dying. Suzanne clamored until the hospital personnel, inexperienced with AIDS and unsympathetic, provided Jim with sufficient morphine to deaden his excruciating pain.

On September 4 Jim died.

"I think that Jim was probably too far down the line when he latched on to the egg lecithin," Kevin commented. "The funny thing was that he stayed stable for so long. Now that Jim's gone, there's a void, and I'm going to have to find some way of filling the time. I have to contribute somehow." (Kevin survived another two years, dying in October 1990.)

Tom Hannan's lover Steve developed a spastic condition and because of pulmonary Karposi's sarcoma was unable to hold down food or medication and had stopped ingesting the egg lecithin. (Steve lingered until January 1988.) All Tom could say about the effect of lecithin on himself was that he was working at the office every day from 9 until late at night.

◆ ◆ ◆

Even before the first distribution by the PWA Health Group, members of the New Jersey Hemophiliac Association had begun to experiment with the egg lecithin variant. An estimated 70 percent of the hemophiliacs in the state had been infected with HIV through contaminated blood.

Mrs. V and her Philadelphia physician saw John James's reprint of the home formula for AL721 in the *AIDS Treatment News*. They decided to experiment with the egg lecithin variant. Two years earlier Mrs. V's eldest son, a hemophiliac, had died of cirrhosis of the liver. Her remaining sons, twins, 26 years of age, were also hemophiliacs. One was crippled in the hand from what is called Wolfman's contraction. He suffered also from arthritis and a bad knee.

In January 1986 Jim, the other twin, came down with persistent eye and ear infections along with a dry cough. The family physician diagnosed it at first as influenza. Mrs. V suspected that he was infected with HIV, and, in fact, in March 1987 Jim came down with pneumocystis carinii pneumonia. Analysis of stored blood showed that Jim had been infected for five years, since 1982. Jim's doctor prescribed bactrim as a prophylaxis against PCP. Jim was hospitalized for twenty-two days. He went from 160 pounds to about 130.

The doctor told Mrs. V that her son's prognosis was not good. "Jim is a fighter, and I don't want to hear that my son is going to die," said Mrs. V. They changed doctors. According to Mrs. V, the new physician—Dr. Stephen Hauptmann of Jefferson University Hospital in Philadelphia—is "wonderful. He's a person first and a doctor second. He goes the way Jim wants to go, with the way Jim wants to be treated. He calls us by first names." In April Dr. Hauptmann put Jim on ten milligrams daily of the AL721 analog home formula. Jim gained thirty pounds in two months. His T4 count went from 60 to 180. He regained his energy and had a general sense of good health. Hauptmann invited Jim to enter a clinical trial with a monthly transfusion of lymphocytes drawn from Mrs. V. His T4 cell count rose as high as 420.

Hauptmann also put Jim on AZT. A full dose brought bad side effects. In April 1988 Jim contracted hepatitis from a medication against hemorrhaging, a frequent problem with hemophiliacs, and Hauptmann took him off all medications. In three weeks he lost fifteen pounds.

◆ ◆ ◆

Self-Empowerment Everywhere!

The yearning for self-empowerment as demonstrated by the New York PWA Health Group was evidenced in a rapid multiplication of distribution and other activist groups around the nation. Common to all groups was the ingenuity, imagination and dedication of the initiators. Each group had a different story to tell—often of people wracked by disease, no longer able to support themselves by regular employment and devoting their final days and last energies to obtaining treatments for themselves and for fellow PWAs.[2]

By the time of the publication of this book, a large percentage of the people mentioned in the following pages had perished.

TULSA, OKLAHOMA

In May 1986, eight months before the founding of the New York PWA Health Group, David Robison, who four years earlier at the age of 27 had been diagnosed as having AIDS Related Complex (ARC), was told that his lover, suffering from full-blown AIDS, had only weeks to live. A friend at a local hospital, researching with the hospital computer, assembled titles of articles on HIV therapies. David sat in the Oklahoma University Medical School library with a medical dictionary at his side and put himself through an intensive course in microbiology, virology and immunology. Photocopying significant articles, he developed extensive files. He started Oklahoma Project Inform and disseminated what he learned.

In treating his dying lover, whom he managed to keep alive for a year, David discovered that by buying products in bulk he could reduce expenditures. In the summer of 1986 he organized Nutrico, a distribution service of alternative therapies. After newspaper articles, a television interview and a report in the San Francisco Project Inform publication, his clientele grew until he developed a file of some 1,500 names, including some 300 active clients in forty-five states as well as in Canada and even in Costa Rica. By December 1987 he was selling a hundred kilos of an AL721 analog a month.

SAN FRANCISCO

In November 1986 John Fox, then 39, noticed a small lesion on his calf. It was Kaposi's sarcoma. A self-proclaimed workaholic with a knack for making money, John had accumulated substantial savings, and upon his diagnosis, he retired. "I decided," he said, "that if I had only X amount of time left, I was going to enjoy it."

In January 1987, John read in John James's *AIDS Treatment News* the home manufacturing formula for AL721. In March John contacted Tom Hannan. When Tom expressed concern about disposing of the 200 kilos of the egg lecithin variant the New York PWA Health Group had ordered from American Roland, John sent a check for $5,000 for twenty-five kilos for distribution in San Francisco.

Fearful of endangering their public funding, no San Francisco organization, John discovered, would sponsor the distribution of an unauthorized substance. John did find a collaborator, however, in Tom O'Connor, a well-known AIDS activist. They assembled some thirty friends and acquaintances and formed Healing Alternatives.

"Since I became involved," said John, "I've been busier than I ever was when I was working. I'm on the telephone constantly."

---

[2] Leaders of many more groups than are represented in this chapter (a small percentage of the total that were organized) were interviewed. Regrettably, only a few of the groups could be included in the final manuscript.

John James agreed to participate in the new organization until it got under way. Joining the board also was a successful business consultant, a PWA, financially able to devote much free time to the group's activities. In New York two men in their early thirties, Peter Esposito with full-blown AIDS and his lover Terry (not his real name) sero-positive but asymptomatic, who were planning to move to San Francisco, learned about Fox's activity from Tom Hannan. Arriving in San Francisco, Terry, an accountant, took charge of the Healing Alternatives accounts; Peter became a part-time director.

In June placards announcing a public meeting were posted in gay neighborhoods, and Fox appeared on television. About 350 people filled the house.

By October Healing Alternatives was in full operation. Every Tuesday at the Metropolitan Community Church, after a business meeting the doors were opened to people lined up to buy an AL721 analog and other alternative therapies.

By December the group was selling fifty kilos of the lecithin variant every Tuesday. By April 1988, operating under a new name, The Healing Alternatives Foundation, the group was selling a hundred kilos a week and was serving 1,000 clients. A headquarters was established in a storefront equipped with an AIDS reference library. The foundation was able to make a $1,500 emergency grant to ACT NOW (AIDS Coalition to Network, Organize and Win—the national organization that had developed out of New York's ACT UP) and joined the PWA Health Group in New York in pledging several thousand dollars to send a physician to Africa to investigate MM-1, a new AIDS therapy developed there.

On August 26, 1988, twenty-two months after his diagnosis as a PWA and after three months of serious illness, John Fox died. In a eulogy in the *AIDS Treatment News*, John James wrote:

> John was a leading organizer and president of the board of the buyers club. . . .
> He had become a leading expert on AIDS treatments, spending much of his
> time on the phone with physicians, scientists, and persons with AIDS
> throughout the United States and beyond. People in San Francisco will
> remember his talks on treatments almost every Tuesday night at meetings of
> Healing Alternatives. . . . John's courage, enthusiasm, and willingness to help
> others will never be forgotten by those who knew him.

In October, two months after John Fox's death, the group lost their director with the death of Peter Esposito.

MINNEAPOLIS

Steven Katz, organizer of the activist group in Minneapolis, declared of the local AIDS service organization, "They are more concerned with death and dying than with living. They provide no support and no empowerment to PWAs."

In 1985 Steven, Betty O'Brian and Paul Loman founded a new organization, The Aliveness Project.

An occupational and recreational therapist, Steven, 42, was diagnosed with Kaposi's sarcoma in 1982. Paul, a 44-year-old factory worker, was diagnosed with

ARC in 1985; in October 1987 he came down with a strange cancer. Betty, a registered nurse who works primarily with children, is in her late thirties. When her brother, who had lived in Steven's house (Steven provided shelter to homeless PWAs), died in 1985, she became active in AIDS programs.

The three friends contacted PWA organizations around the country to find out what others were doing, set up a speakers' bureau to give talks on "Living with AIDS," formed a weekly support group and began visiting hospitalized PWAs. Next they turned to making alternative treatments available, starting with vitamins and herbs.

"We provide information," said Steven, "regarding what is available and encourage people to go on protocols if they are interested in buying a product. We even provide money for the first month's supply, money we obtain from private contributions." (Aliveness established good relations with a cross-section of the city's population, gay and straight, black and white, and of all ethnic groups.)

By late 1987, two years after the founding of the Aliveness Project, a governing board of thirty was meeting once a month, each member holding a particular responsibility. Almost all board members were PWAs or PWARCs. Aliveness had no clients, only people involved in its projects. Volunteers, primarily PWAs, were assigned to people who requested buddy assistance.

During the first two years of Aliveness's existence the speakers' bureau was enlarged, and speakers were provided to hospitals, religious organizations and schools. Aliveness assisted hospitals throughout the state in setting up AIDS care programs. The organization published a newsletter dealing with alternate approaches to AIDS and pamphlets directed to the newly diagnosed and their families.

The support groups increased from one to twelve per week, including one for children, each with an average attendance of thirty-five and forty-five people. Programs were developed for caregivers and for clergy. A meal was served to PWAs once a week at an interdenominational church.

In the fall of 1987 Aliveness participated actively in a six-day Minnesota state conference on AIDS. "People," reported Steven, "prefer to hear us rather than professionals."

Word of the success of Aliveness spread beyond the state. *Life* magazine came to interview the leaders early in December 1987. The group was also featured on national television on "Nightline," and the program "West 57th Street" included Aliveness in a story on adolescents and AIDS. "What the media like about us," explains Steven, "is that we're Mid-America. Also we believe in choice, no right or wrong way."

Tom O'Connor of the San Francisco group convinced the leaders of Aliveness of the potential usefulness of AL721. Aliveness encouraged individuals to order on their own, for it was Aliveness policy to encourage initiative among PWAs, to develop in each a sense of helping himself.

SAN DIEGO

Tom Hansen was born in Albany, Illinois. He majored in international relations at the University of Colorado at Boulder and then studied international management at the graduate school of the University of Arizona. In 1986 he obtained a position as purchasing agent for the San Diego Community College. In January 1987 he was diagnosed as having ARC.

Tom first learned about the egg lecithin variant upon seeing Steve Gavin's home formula in the *New York Native*. Seven PWAs met at Tom's home on May 8, 1987 and formed the Alliance 7 Buyers Club. They sought the collaboration of Healing Alternatives in San Francisco.

By the summer Tom found himself shouldering the entire responsibility except, briefly, when he was assisted by a former architect, a PWARC. Accepted in 1986 into a clinical test of Ribavirin, this man was one of those who received a placebo. Contracting PCP, he was given no medication (so as not to upset a clinical test in which he was enrolled). He came down with retinitis in his eyes, and a catheter was implanted in him for treatment of cytomegalovirus, a frequent opportunistic disease with HIV.

In September, having lost his collaborator, Tom turned the operation into a for-profit business. As of December 1987 he was ordering about fifteen kilos of egg lecithin a month, charging a small markup over the wholesale price.

Tom himself experienced all the classic symptoms of a PWARC—a mouth infection, night sweats, candidiasis and swollen lymph glands as well as a lung infection that for forty-five days did not respond to antibiotics. After taking the AL721 analog, he says, all his symptoms disappeared. "I consider it," Tom says, "the foundation block of my well being. I call egg lecithin the insulin for AIDS. The average human cell lives for seven years, and I hope that if I continue to take the egg lecithin for seven years, the last infected cell will die."

Tom participated in an hour-long radio talk show with two local physicians. He was interviewed by NBC television news, and on October 22, 1987 the *Philadelphia Inquirer* included him in a report about PWAs around the nation in a segment headed "A victim treats himself." The article described Tom as "a 31-year-old man with a square jaw, upturned nose and deep brown eyes. . . . By 1983, he was an alcoholic, a serious drug user and a frequenter of the gay bar scene. AIDS has changed all that," the article stated. "Hansen has quit cigarettes, alcohol and drugs. He gets plenty of sleep, exercises every day, prays, and tries to imagine good things for himself."

Of himself the article quoted Tom as saying: "I am a shining example of someone who is recovering. I think it important to let people know that they can take these things into their own hands in personal health management. I have gone through six doctors. Most of them knew less than I."

LONG BEACH, CALIFORNIA

At 29, Ron Parron, a high school graduate from Orlando, Florida, could look back upon a Horatio Alger career. At the McDonald's food chain he worked his way up from janitor to executive by the age of 19. Subsequently, he held an administrative position at General Mills and in the Jack in the Box chain. At the age of 25, however, he began to experience subtle changes in his body. After suffering candidiasis and lymphadenopathy so acute that his left eardrum burst, Ron was diagnosed with ARC. He developed ulcers in his esophagus and was given acute antacid therapy and constrictors for his esophagus and stomach muscles. He suffered terrible chest pains. He began taking AZT, acyclovir, an antidepressant as well as an AL721 analog. For about two weeks he had diarrhea from the egg lecithin. "I called the doctor today and said, 'I've got to do something. I haven't slept for four nights.'"

Late in 1986 from Project Inform in San Francisco Ron obtained directions for mixing DNCB, a topical agent employed as an alternate therapy by people infected with HIV. Producing a larger quantity than he needed, he called Project Inform and asked what he should do with the surplus. He was told that someone was needed in the Long Beach area to distribute therapeutic substances. Ron agreed to accept the responsibility, and Project Inform published his telephone number and arranged newspaper and television interviews for him.

Working out of his home, Ron began distributing "many things, too many, including vitamins, minerals and herbs." The *Los Angeles Times* ran a long article about his enterprise. At the end of 1987 Ron directed his effort primarily to the distribution of an AL721 analog, ordering twenty to thirty kilos a month. When the business expanded he bought a computer. His apartment was broken into, and the computer along with his burglar alarm were stolen.

Ron had no family. "In the holiday time," he said, "it's hard. All I have is people pulling at me in all directions." No longer employed, he had to wait a long time before his application for social security was approved. He reduced his living expenses to a minimum.

ORLANDO, FLORIDA

Jim Sammone, a PWA in his early thirties, was the catalyst in Orlando, where by the end of 1987 there were an estimated 200 individuals seriously ill with HIV infection. Until July 1987 Jim served as a public relations person for Centaur (Central Florida AIDS Unified Resources), an organization with 200 members. He became discouraged with the timidity of the leaders of the organization and with what he considered to be an exaggerated concern about their public image.

Suffering from acute lymphoma, Jim could not waste time in organizational conflicts. Nor was he emotionally suited for involvement in providing services to PWAs; he bore too much grief from the loss of close friends. On the other hand, he was eager to participate in the kind of activism of the PWA Coalition in New York, Project Inform in San Francisco and other groups throughout the country. Jim contacted John Fascuti, a PWA with a similar desire for an activist approach to the epidemic.

In 1985, then 30, John, a competitive athlete while at the University of Florida and a successful real estate broker, was diagnosed as HIV-positive. He traveled to Mexico to buy Ribavirin and isoprinosine. "I believe that my aggressiveness," he says, "saved my life." John contacted individuals and organizations in the national AIDS network, including Project Inform, and learned of other therapies.

At an organizational meeting of some ten people in August 1987, John offered the New York PWA Coalition as a model for the new Orlando group, AIDS Coalition Endowment (ACE). Jim was elected president; John, vice-president. John, who had been taking an AL721 analog since ordering a quantity at the first distribution by the New York PWA Health Group in May, took charge of the distribution of the substance. He introduced a novel payment system under which purchasers who were employed or otherwise capable of paying full price were charged above the wholesale price, while those of limited means were charged half-price and the indigent were given an allotment at no cost.

Miriam Saunders, 32, co-founder of a local theater, accepted the major responsibility for fundraising for ACE. "I was finding myself constantly going to memorial services," she reports. "How long can you go around simply grieving? Jim Sammone and I hit it off immediately," says Miriam, and she joined Jim in organizing ACE. In October 1987 they held a fundraising jazz concert at which they raised $6,000. Thereafter the group planned further fundraisers to establish a hospice for dying PWAs.

Miriam, John and Jim all spoke with respect and affection of one of their main collaborators, Lois Adams. A licensed consultant pharmacist and president of Home Health Care Services, Inc., whose officers include the commander of the 14th Fleet Naval Hospital, Lois had served as president of the Florida Pharmacy Association and was a member of the University of Florida College of Health Advisory Board as well as the board of Central Florida AIDS Resources and the AIDS Task Force of the University of Central Florida. "When some very fine people you know die of AIDS, you become committed," Lois declared. "It affects not only the gay community, it affects everybody."

In May 1987 John showed Lois the AL721 analog he had obtained from the PWA Health Group. In December 1987, after debating whether to manufacture the egg lecithin variant ("I didn't want to invest in a chicken farm"), she placed an initial order for 600 kilos.

In early December when Jim was interviewed on the telephone, he sounded full of life. At the end of the month, however, he was hospitalized and in great pain. Upon opening him up, the surgeons discovered that he was clogged with toxic waste built up from the AZT he had been taking. There was nothing they could do. He died on January 2, 1988.

Jim's mother entered activity at ACE, seeking to replace her son.

A year later John Fascuti died.

CHICAGO

In his mid-thirties, Chris Clason had been a theater arts major at Eastern Michigan University, an actor and entertainer and a caterer as well as an employee of the Federal Environmental Protection Agency.

In January 1986 exploratory surgery revealed next to one of Chris's kidneys a cluster of swollen lymph glands causing a blockage and forcing lymphatic fluid to drain into his left leg, which puffed up like a balloon. In February 1987 he took an antibodies test and discovered that he was HIV-positive.

Chris applied for membership in an ARC support group. Informed that the cost would be $75 per session, Chris wrote a prospectus for a group of his own which eventually would come to be called Test Positive Aware (TPA). In March 1987 Chris called a planning meeting. To the sixteen people who responded to a notice in a local gay publication, Chris described the need for an "aggressive, ambitious and progressive collection of individuals who are exploring the many aspects and impacts of healthy living with HIV infection."

In addition to weekly meetings for the discussion of topics of interest to people with HIV infection, TPA held monthly after-meeting socials at the homes of members. It published a newsletter and fact sheets and began developing a resource directory. The September newsletter declared proudly: "Thanks to the input, energy and interest of its membership, TPA is fast becoming one of the most comprehensive and thorough information networks on issues that affect HIV-impacted people in the Midwest, if not the country." It noted, too: "We have learned that there is more to life than T-cell counts alone. We are discovering inner strengths and the courage to face head-on all aspects of HIV infection."

At a December meeting Chris reported a membership approaching 130 and the receipt of a donation of $1,000 from a man whose lover had died of AIDS with which TPA would publish an official brochure dedicated to the memory of the donor's lover. Chris also announced that TPA was about to move into its own offices and that a second meeting would be held each week with the possibility even of a third.

By December up to thirty members had been using the egg lecithin variant for at least two months. Most reported an increase in energy; some, a reduced swelling of lymph glands and relief from other minor symptoms.

Plans were developed to print forms and questionnaires to monitor the health status of those using an AL721 analog.

VANCOUVER, CANADA

The self-empowerment movement in the United States inspired PWAs across the border. With a population about equal to California's, Canada at the end of 1987 had registered fewer cases of AIDS (approximately 1,400) than the city of San Francisco. Some 300 were concentrated in Vancouver. "It is very easy," says Kevin Brown, 38, an elementary school teacher and a founder of the Vancouver PWA Coalition, "for our government to declare it a minor disease and to put little effort into combatting it." On the other hand, according to Kevin, "the excitement in the United States has generated fear and hysteria in Canada."

After a mention in the *New York Native*, the Coalition, the only PWA activist organization in Canada, began receiving telephone calls from across Canada, and the members began discussing ways to promote activity elsewhere.

On June 5, 1985 Kevin was diagnosed as having PCP. "The next day," he relates, "I decided that crying was boring and that I'd better get on with my life. I've been active ever since, and maybe that's helped me to live these two and a half years." Kevin continued to teach after his diagnosis until his health deteriorated to an obvious degree. "I hold the PCP record in Vancouver," he declares, "six bouts in two and a half years."

According to Kevin an activist organization was necessary because the province of British Columbia, administered by an ultraconservative political party, had no use for gays or for any people with alternate life styles. "They feel," declares Kevin, "that those who have AIDS deserved to get it in the first place." The province preached abstinence as the answer to the plague. Municipal legislation in Vancouver permitted medical officers to quarantine and isolate "irresponsible persons" with AIDS.

AIDS Vancouver, the establishment gay organization, conducted education and support programs for PWAs but rejected activist protest. "We have the sense," says Kevin, "that very little would be done unless PWAs had a very vocal presence and stood up for their rights." In 1985 Kevin was joined by Warren Hansen, an accountant in his early thirties, and Paavi Nirvela, a construction worker (who died in the fall of 1987), in forming the Vancouver PWA Coalition. In the spring of 1986 Kevin and his friends organized a march on the British Columbia provincial legislature, their first major action. The fifteen demonstrators were outnumbered by the representatives of the media.

The Coalition held regular meetings, some of which attracted as many as ninety people. Anyone who had AIDS was considered a member. The Coalition was run by a nine-member board and had two staff members, one full-time and one part-time. It maintained an office as well as a "living room," a social meeting space like the one operated by the PWA Coalition in New York.

The city administration proved helpful. "We're doing a lot of social work for them," explained Kevin. "We visit people in the hospitals, we hold support group meetings." The Coalition offered training seminars for the Vancouver school board and conducted a speakers' bureau.

Partly as a result of strenuous lobbying by the Coalition, AZT was made available in Canada as an experimental therapy. The Canadian federal government was not, however, exploring alternative therapies. "We seem to have very few researchers in Canada," says Kevin, "who are willing to look into AIDS therapies. Most of the doctors on the front lines are so overworked and burned out that they don't have energy or time to investigate other substances."

In June 1987, on his way to the IIIrd International AIDS Conference in Washington, where he was one of the speakers, Kevin conferred with leaders of the PWA Health Group. Returning to Vancouver, he and his associates investigated the documentation on AL721 and decided to "give it a go." The Coalition's board voted to fund a study with ten people for a six-month period under the supervision of a local oncologist. Initial blood work was done, to be followed by monthly reports. As of December 1987, thirty people were taking an AL721 analog.

When Kevin called a news conference and announced over national television that the Coalition was initiating the first patient-organized research project in Canada, the Coalition began receiving telephone calls from across Canada. The *Vancouver Sun* for September 25, 1987 quoted Kevin as saying:

> The message we want to send to the public and to the government is that people with AIDS are part of the solution, not just the problem. We want others to start taking an active part in getting more research going. If we waited for the federal government to become more serious about research into AIDS therapy we'd all be dead before they started.

At an international AIDS symposium in Ottawa, a federal official warned Kevin: "We're more than aware of your study. We know that you bring in the egg lecithin as a food product. The minute you administer it as a medical treatment, it comes under the jurisdiction of the Health Protection Branch. Since you do not have our permission to carry out this supposed medical treatment, we can shut you down."

"You will have your first PWA riot," Kevin responded. "It would be political suicide for you."

(On February 26, 1989 the *New York Times* reported: "The Canadian Government has sent out notices to every doctor in Canada that it will allow patients with life-threatening diseases to obtain any drugs companies are willing to sell, even if no country has approved the drugs for marketing." The *Times* quoted Michael Callen, the New York PWA activist, as commenting that the policy "starkly demonstrates that in Canada they're prepared to view AIDS as an emergency. This should embarrass the FDA. It should light a fire under them.")

LONDON, ENGLAND

On a visit to New York in March 1987, Colin Clark learned of the plans of the PWA Health Group to distribute an AL721 analog. Upon returning home, Colin discussed what he had learned with leaders of Frontliners, an English counterpart to the PWA Coalition, and found them sympathetic to a similar action with an AL721 analog.

Colin and three friends—two of them PWAs, one in the pharmaceutical business and the other active in gay politics—set up a not-for-profit company, Vanmount Ltd., to import the egg lecithin variant. "By the time it gets through trials [for official authorization]," said Colin, "it's going to be too late. Friends are dying."

Early in June Vanmount received the first two kilos from Germany and assigned them to two PWAs. The group planned a trial with about ten people who were seriously ill. Colin said of one PWA after a month on the egg lecithin variant, "I have never seen such a transformation." Of the other, who had been very seriously ill, it was difficult to tell whether the lecithin was having any effect. "We gave it to him," Colin noted, "because we felt it would be impossible not to give it to him."

By late October Vanmount was supplying about forty people with the egg lecithin variant. Colin himself and one of his associates were taking their product, which they call VM1.

BERLIN, GERMAN FEDERAL REPUBLIC

The Deutsche AIDS-Hilfe is an example of an impressive gay initiative on a national scale. Inaugurated in the spring of 1983 by three men—Gerd Paul, Juergen Roland and Ian Schaefer—by the time it was registered in December 1985 as a national not-for-profit organization it was serving as the parent organization of approximately 75 local AIDS-Hilfe groups ranging in size from 10 to 200 members for a total membership of 4,000, some locals with an employed staff, others run by some of the 3,000 volunteers.

The central office in Berlin had a subscribing membership of 350 organizations and individuals. In addition to a board of directors that included two physicians, the organization had thirty-five employees. Since 1985 it had received federal grants ranging from DM 300,000 in 1985 to DM 2 million in 1986 to DM 5 million in 1987. (A mark was then roughly equivalent to half a dollar.) In addition it collected in membership fees and donations DM 100,000 in 1986 and DM 300,000 in 1987.

The Berlin office was responsible for national education campaigns directed at various target groups, for developing educational materials and for training of volunteers and staff workers at meetings, seminars and workshops. In 1987 AIDS-Hilfe published approximately 10 million pieces of educational materials—brochures, leaflets, posters, stickers and pamphlets—directed to gays, IV drug users, prostitutes, prison inmates, educators, public employees and to the general public. In addition, it conducted a nonprofit distribution of about 250,000 "special" condoms to gays.

In 1987 sixty-six national training programs were conducted, and a media package consisting of three videos along with textbooks directed specifically at "buddies" was produced.

The burgeoning of self-empowerment initiatives throughout the United States as well as in other countries helped set an environment in the United States for the struggle by the AIDS community to prod lethargic and diffident national, state and local administrations into action against the crisis.

By 1989 it was estimated that more than 500 PWA organizations of varying memberships and programs were active throughout the United States.

CHAPTER 9

Ethigen at Bay

Early in 1985 Terry Beirn, a public relations man, joined the staff of the newly organized American Foundation for AIDS Research. A go-getter with boundless self-assurance, Beirn urged Arnold Lippa to prepare a protocol for a clinical test of AL721 in anticipation of the appearance of the Gallo letter. As a result of Beirn's prodding of the FDA Investigation Review Board, approval of the Investigational New Drug (IND) application for a Phase II clinical trial (a Phase I trial tests merely for toxicity) "to evaluate the antiviral and immunologic effects of AL721" was granted in January 1986, within a mere two months.

The protocol called for eleven test patients at St. Luke's/Roosevelt Hospital, a teaching hospital associated with Columbia University, along with two additional overseas groups of equal number, one in London supervised by Anthony Pinching and another in Israel under Zwi Bentwich. In February 1987 the first steps for a trial were initiated at St. Luke's/Roosevelt under the supervision of Drs. Michael H. Grieco and Michael Lange. Only eight asymptomatic patients with Persistent Generalized Lymphadenopathy (PGL, an early stage of the HIV infection) were screened out of forty volunteers.

With postponement of the test month after month because of Ethigen's failure to provide a quantity of AL721, the volunteers, anxious at their HIV infection and yearning for a cure, became angry and despondent, and the physicians, too, were demoralized. (Although Krsek at Houba, Inc. was producing 80 kilos of AL721 a month until ordered to stop in May 1987 and thereafter held in storage 320 kilos awaiting payment, the tests projected in London and Israel as well as that at St. Luke's/Roosevelt were held up on the pretext of a lack of AL721.)

Finally, in July, after six months of dawdling, Lippa asked Krsek, with whom he had previously broken relations, to produce a supply of AL721 on an emergency basis. Krsek recommenced production immediately, and the St. Luke's/Roosevelt test started a month later.

After eight weeks during which the St. Luke's patients were given twenty grams of AL721 daily, Ethigen announced a 60 percent reduction in levels of reverse transcriptase (a biological marker for the presence of the virus), improvement in immune functions and "the first demonstration in humans of any drug showing anti-viral activity . . . [without] any adverse side effects."

Although upon the conclusion of the test one of the patients, consistently uncooperative in following instructions, died, his death did not undermine the morale of the patients and the physicians.

Plans were made to resume the test. With another inexplicable delay of five months, however, the seven remaining patients and the physicians once again experienced a sense of frustration.

One of those who entered the clinical study with great expectations was Dann O'Connor, a dancer in his early thirties. Upon the death of his lover in 1983, Dann was tested as sero-positive. Michael Lange, his physician, prescribed no medication since Dann was asymptomatic except for a slight swelling of his lymph glands. Invited to participate in the St. Luke's/Roosevelt study, Dann reported once a week for tests. At the end of the eight weeks, although encouraged by the restrained optimism of the physicians supervising the study, Dann was not confident that he had found the miracle cure he was seeking. In January 1988, while waiting for the study to resume, Dann came down with a bout of pneumocystis carinii pneumonia. Although the attack was extraordinarily mild, he was now diagnosed as having full-blown AIDS, a development that depressed both the physicians and the other patients in the study. Dann himself did not believe that his illness evidenced the inefficacy of AL721. That winter, in addition to holding down a full-time job, he was "running himself ragged" fundraising for the Martha Graham dance group, of which he had formerly been a member.

In 1978, then 27, Toby, another participant in the clinical test, participated in a series of gay jet set "Red, White and Blue" parties. Originating in San Francisco, the parties, each lasting over a three-day weekend, moved on to Los Angeles, Houston, New Orleans, Atlanta, Washington, New York City, and finally Fire Island. The partygoers took drugs and engaged in what Toby describes as "crazy sex." In New York he lived with one of the first men to contract AIDS. In the late 1970s and early 1980s a hepatitis epidemic was raging in the gay community of New York, and Toby, along with many of the other Red, White and Blue crowd, was one of the victims. He subsequently contracted herpes as well.

Toby settled in New York, a prosperous architect. In 1983 and 1984 he suffered burnout from his fast life style and experienced depression and chronic fevers. He suspected that he was infected with HIV, but his physician advised against taking the test. He began having memory problems. At last, in 1985, he was tested as sero-positive. "If my doctor had had me take the test two years earlier," he says, "I could have done something about it."

Interviewed for the St. Luke's/Roosevelt study in September 1985 Toby experienced a nightmare at the delay until the following summer. In October 1986, however, when the patients were taken off the AL721, Toby felt in good shape. Once again, however, he experienced the frustration of inexplicable delays in the resumption of the test. As the weeks passed, Toby's condition deteriorated.

In February Dann, Toby and the five others were readmitted to a higher-dosage clinical study for a period of six months, a study that was later expanded to a full year. Although after two months "five of the six HIV-positive patients had lower levels of virus in their blood, as measured by the reduction in levels of RT [and] improved immune system response was again observed," in the fall of 1987, abruptly, a second patient died, of PCP.

"I became paranoid," Toby said. "My T cell count declined disastrously. I fell into a depression. We were all disappointed. I'm no longer enthusiastic about AL721. I gambled a lot on this study and put a lot of faith and energy into it. Now I have lost faith. Of course, the experience was made worse by the frustrations we suffered with Praxis [Ethigen]."

◆ ◆ ◆

According to Michael Lange, one of the administrators of the AL721 test, in five of the seven patients in the St. Luke's/Roosevelt study there was a significant, if not total, reduction of the virus; but during the five-month hiatus between the first and second stages of the study the virus reappeared in four of the five within about eight weeks. Four to eight weeks later two patients advanced toward a real AIDS condition—one came down with PCP and one with lymphoma. Since the number of patients was so small, it was possible that these developments represented mere coincidence.

Lange was concerned at any discontinuance of treatment with AL721. He noted that with lupus, a viral disease with some similarity to AIDS, discontinuance of steroid therapy leads to a rebound effect. (Indeed, Shinitzky had found in his testing of geriatric patients that termination of AL721 resulted in a relapse in their immune systems.)

On the other hand, Lange had personal knowledge of PWAs on AZT who lost so many red cells as to need two or three transfusions within four months. With the administration of AL721 they no longer required transfusions. Nevertheless, he was of the opinion that not enough was known to distinguish among those patients who showed a remarkable positive response to AL721, those who showed a minor positive reaction and those who showed no positive effect at all. Like many other physicians, Lange noted that some patients gain an almost immediate sense of well-being from the treatment. AL721 seemed to have an antiviral as well as an anti-inflammatory effect, he said, but the question was whether in the suppression of the virus the progression of the disease was halted.

Lange had a special problem in judging AL721 inasmuch as he questioned whether HIV was actually the cause of AIDS. "We know patients who have been infected for six or seven years without falling ill or showing any decline in their immune systems." Years before people became ill, Lange noted, it was possible to detect surrogate factors that produce or indicate chronic inflammatory conditions. Cells, including some without infected receptors, were destroyed through an immune reaction, a chronic inflammatory reaction. It might well have been that by the time a patient advanced to ARC or AIDS the virus which had started the process was no longer needed to continue it.

Clinical Tests Held and Not Held

Foreign scientists who contracted with Praxis to conduct experiments were as chagrined at the company's procrastination and neglect as the thousands of PWAs who eagerly awaited large-scale production of AL721.

At the regional hospital at Clermont-Ferrand in France, Dr. Labbe, a short, bespectacled man, all business, had little time to spare for an interview. At the mention of Meir Shinitzky's name, however, he picked up the telephone and called in Dr. Claude Motta, an associate with whom he had performed clinical tests with AL721 with children suffering from cystic fibrosis, a painful and widespread disease in which mucous blocks the lungs and digestive system. (Motta had previously worked with Shinitzky on mucous analysis at the Weizmann Institute.) In 1983 in an initial study of AL721 formulated into a spray, he and Labbe achieved promising results in loosening mucous blockage.

In 1985 Lippa sent David A. Scheer, a Praxis consultant,[1] to ask Labbe and Motta to conduct another intensive test. Accordingly, in 1986 they administered AL721 to a group of five children and adolescents suffering from cystic fibrosis. The patients tolerated the AL721 well, suffered no adverse side effects and registered an improvement in expectoration.

The two physicians were indignant at receiving no acknowledgment of the report they dispatched to the United States and no replies to subsequent letters. Furthermore, they were chagrined at having to abandon a promising investigation because of Ethigen's failure to furnish additional supplies of AL721. "The only material we have been able to obtain," they declared, "we have received from Skornik in Israel."

In a covering letter to an abstract of the results of their studies Labbe described their investigation as "a brief study from which one cannot draw any decisive conclusions regarding the effect of AL721 on mucous viscosity. We would very much like to conduct a controlled study with a much larger number of patients and over a period of at least a year. I hope that will soon be possible."

---

[1] Scheer runs a consulting firm in New Haven, Connecticut, and holds a part-time position at the Yale Medical School. Lippa had included his name among the signers of the letter to the *New England Journal of Medicine*. Scheer was granted the privilege of purchasing company options at one cent per share. He would answer no questions regarding his association with Ethigen.

In January 1986, after an approach from Lippa, Anthony Pinching of St. Mary's Hospital Medical School in London obtained approval from the United Kingdom Department of Health and Social Services to hold a clinical trial of AL721 with patients infected with HIV. In a letter in July 1987 Pinching expressed his chagrin that eighteen months after having formulated plans for a clinical trial, he was still confronting difficulty in obtaining supplies of AL721. "I suggest," he wrote, "that you discuss matters relating to any planned trials or distribution with Praxis/Ethigen."

◆ ◆ ◆

In the fall of 1987, recognizing that much time might elapse before large-scale, multicentered clinical studies of AL721 would be initiated in the United States, Meir Shinitzky, Yehuda Skornik, Israel Yust and V. Zakut, a colleague of Skornik's at Rokach Hospital, felt compelled to issue a preliminary report of results of administration of AL721 to a mere six AIDS and four ARC patients involved in "a compassionate open trial," out of the forty-three whom they had treated. Of the ten patients in the report, one had been taking AL721 since April 1986 (Michael May); one, since November 1986; four, since December 1986; one, since January 1987; and three since February 1987. They reported "a gradual improvement in the overt clinical state after two weeks of treatment" in most patients; a significant improvement in all patients after three months, including decline in body temperature among those who suffered from chronic fever; a 90 percent reduction in viral level after twelve weeks in three patients; and a recovery approaching normal leukocyte in four patients after three months of treatment. In addition, a significant improvement "in general feeling and body function" had been observed among almost all the patients, three of whom had previously been considered terminal. None of the ten patients displayed any major infection after three months of treatment. They recommended that an immune stimulant be added after three months of AL721 treatment and suggested that AL721 might "also act as an adjuvant in combination with other anti-viral drugs (e.g. AZT)."

The report did not impress the delegates either as far as the number of patients or the results were concerned.

Zwi Bentwich of Kaplan Hospital did not participate in drafting the study. Of the twenty or so patients he had had over the previous year, two showed an improvement in T4 cell count, decrease of fever and increased weight. Two had died. He was about to commence a clinical trial with seventeen PGL and borderline ARC patients with negative antigen count and lowered immunity. Meanwhile, he was holding his judgment of AL721 in abeyance.

Ethigen Bankrupt

From its initial formation as a corporate entity, Jacobson's firm showed an annual deficit. Even in June 1985, after obtaining more than $3.5 million from a public stock offering, the firm's net loss totaled $1,346,126. In the fall of 1985, at the time of the publication of the Gallo letter in the *New England Journal of Medicine*, with no product for sale and ever-mounting annual deficits, Praxis was unable to renew a $20 million liability insurance policy or to obtain more than $500,000 in insurance for its clinical trials.

By June 1987 the firm's net loss had grown to $6,296,314, and working capital on hand amounted to only $156,000. In a July 1987 submission to the Securities and Exchange Commission (SEC), Ethigen (the name was changed from Praxis in May 1987) officials admitted that the company did not "possess the financial, technical and other resources necessary to conduct and complete the required testing and procedures necessary to obtain governmental approval to market AL721 as an ethical pharmaceutical, or to conduct research and development related to the Company's existing biotechnology products." They estimated that the company would "deplete its cash reserves by September 1987." Even if FDA did eventually grant authorization for the sale of AL721 as an ethical pharmaceutical, the company could not be certain that it would be "economically feasible to commercialize AL721."

In August 1987, to meet the crisis threatening Ethigen's continued existence, the corporation applied to SEC to hold a public stock offering of $6.5 million. For interim financing, notes were issued for $1 million at 10.5 percent interest to be redeemed upon the holding of the stock offering or on March 31, 1988, whichever occurred sooner. Jacobson subscribed to 25 percent of the notes; Lippa, to 5 percent.

Early in November Linda Hunt called John James for an appointment for herself and "Jake." Hunt arrived some days later but in the company of a man named Rosenberg, a Los Angeles public relations man. They informed James that confronting imminent bankruptcy Jacobson had decided to release AL721 as a food supplement for sale in health-food stores and elsewhere. They sought James's cooperation in publicizing their forthcoming over-the-counter product.

On November 10 Tom Hannan received a call from a Bill Meeseheimer, who said he was employed at the American Foundation for AIDS Research (AmFAR) in Los Angeles. He explained, however, that he was not calling for AmFAR but rather for a friend—Linda Hunt, Ethigen's publicity director. Recalling Tom's impassioned but fruitless appeal to Jacobson six months earlier for assistance in the PWA Health Group's distribution of an egg lecithin variant, Hunt apparently feared she would receive an unfriendly reception if she called directly. Through this AmFAR acquaintance she sought to find out the marketing prospects for the new Ethigen product.

Hunt also asked Martin Delaney, director of Project Inform, to raise with FDA Commissioner Frank Young the question of the difference between AL721 and the various egg lecithin products being distributed throughout the country. The company, Hunt told Delaney, had recently completed tests of eight variants of AL721 produced in New York City. She promised to inform Delaney promptly of the results. After days passed without a call, Delaney telephoned and asked for the information forthwith. "Whether it helps or hurts," Delaney declared, "I want to get this out to the community."

"That would be very helpful," replied an apparently grateful Hunt. "I didn't know how to publicize these findings myself." Hunt never called Delaney.

Weeks later Delaney learned that months earlier the New York PWA Health Group had, indeed, submitted eight samples of AL721 analogs to Lippa for testing. Lippa rejected the six samples the PWA group knew to be unsatisfactory and found the other two acceptable.

"Our Responsibility to Our Shareholders"

Jacobson and Lippa had rejected another alternative for avoiding a collapse of their corporation, a rejection that would cost them dearly. In July, impressed with what he heard and read about the egg lecithin variant, Stephen Levine, a successful entrepreneur and a scientist of some standing, telephoned Jacobson with an offer to produce and distribute AL721 for Ethigen.

Shortly after obtaining his doctorate in genetics and molecular biology, Levine came down with environmental illness, suffering severe reactions to foods and chemicals. Experimenting with various treatments, he cured himself. Out of this experience he developed a book on free radical chemistry, a book subsequently translated into several languages. In addition, he founded Nutri-Cology, Inc., a health-food distribution firm at San Leandro, near San Francisco.

In a meeting with Jacobson and Jacobson's associate Robert N. Weingarten in Ethigen's Los Angeles office, Levine confronted them with their Catch 22 situation. "You have something that may work," he said, "and you're not selling it, and you're preventing it from being sold." Jacobson and Weingarten shrugged. Their first responsibility, they declared, was to their stockholders. (Levine had studied the Ethigen submissions to SEC and was aware not only of their financial circumstances but also that Jacobson held approximately one-third of the corporation's shares and that Weingarten was another major stockholder.) They were convinced, they said, that the pursuit of FDA authorization of AL721 as an ethical pharmaceutical was the more profitable route for their shareholders.

Levine decided that in Jacobson he was confronting what he calls "a regular Los Angeles type," suave and unpredictable. He suspected that in any business arrangement Jacobson and Weingarten would demand excessive royalties. Working with them, he concluded, would pose too many difficulties. He arranged with a pharmaceutical manufacturer with whom he had long had connections to develop a formula for large-scale production of an AL721 analog with a close approximation to the 7:2:1 proportions. Levine quickly won a sizable share of the AL721 market.

In Place of Ethigen

But Stephen Levine was not among the first to enter the competition for the AL721 market.

EGGSACT

As early as 1983 Bill Powell and two friends, all employed in the health-food industry, began research in nutrition. Creatures of the sixties, Bill, 35, was a college dropout; one of his associates was a high school dropout; and the other had a degree as a computer programmer. Inspired by John James's articles about AL721, Bill and his two friends studied Shinitzky's reports and then discussed with James the possibility of developing a 7:2:1 product from PC-55, a commercial egg lecithin product. John urged Bill and his colleagues to produce an AL721 analog as soon as possible.

On April 1, 1987, after a year of preparation, under the company name Intrend, they began distribution of their own product, EggsAct—Activated Egg Lecithin— the first AL721 analog available commercially in the United States. In the fall of 1987 Skornik, unable to obtain a sufficient quantity of material from Shinitzky, ordered EggsAct for some of his patients. In October Bill and his associates contributed a quantity of the product to Australia to Dr. Julian Gold, director of an AIDS center in Sydney, for a clinical study to begin in January 1988. A hemophiliac support group in northern California asked their assistance in setting up a small study at Stanford Medical Center. By late 1987 a health-food distributor had placed EggsAct in more than 300 health stores throughout the United States.

JARROW FORMULAS

"How can you raise five and a half million dollars for an R & D corporation," Jarrow Rogovin exclaimed about Ethigen, "spend three and a half million, snarl at everybody that they're violating some patent, and meantime where has all the money gone? On a shoe string I have become the country's largest distributor of egg lecithin, and I think I'm saving lives. Jacobson's incompetence has provided me with a wonderful business and a community service opportunity."

Learning about egg lecithin from the John James newsletter, Rogovin found a German manufacturer to produce the lecithin variant. This product did not match those of other manufacturers in achieving the 7:2:1 ratio and contained a proportion of the less expensive soy lecithin, but Rogovin, an aggressive salesman, offered it at a lower price than his competitors. He quoted Meir Shinitzky as saying that there was no difference between the two. In fact, Shinitzky declared that because of the similarity of egg yolk to the human cell, egg lecithin might well be more effective.

AMERICAN ROLAND

Tom Hannan rejoiced at finding this source for the first PWA Health Group distribution of the egg lecithin variant. Mel Blum, the vice president and chief scientist at American Roland, insisted that his firm would not accept any orders from the PWA Health Group if Tom continued to make medical claims for the compound. He had difficulty in persuading Tom about some of the scientific problems involved in developing an acceptable product. Factors like cholesterol content and the kind of cholesterol, he declared, and the amount of residual solvents were important in establishing a lecithin of pharmaceutical quality. Concerned solely with the 7:2:1 proportions, Tom, on the other hand, was frustrated at his apparent difficulty in convincing Blum of the importance of this factor.

A small, inexpensive analytical laboratory used by the PWA Health Group claimed that the American Roland product PE (one of the three components of AL721) level was only about 5 or 6 percent (as against an "ideal" 10 percent). Blum retorted that the people at the laboratory had no conception of double bonding of a molecule and did not understand that without the HPLC method (High Performance Liquid Chromatography) employed by American Roland they were incapable of achieving a precise analysis of his product. "The lab's method is the one used in Israel," Tom replied. (Meir Shinitzky subsequently admitted that the HPLC method of analysis was superior to the one he had been using. He lacked the equipment for it.)

Although the New York and the San Francisco distribution groups found less expensive sources for analogs, American Roland continued to market its product.

HOUBA, INC.

In 1983 George Krsek, president of Houba and a biochemist with long experience as a research pharmacist, developed the formula for large-scale manufacture of AL721 for Ethigen (with Shinitzky in attendance as a consultant) and thereafter provided the AL721 for clinical tests beginning in that year and continuing through the ATEU tests of 1987. Over the years Krsek had been disturbed at the delay in production of AL721 for general distribution. "There are a lot of people out there suffering," said Krsek. "If AL721 is helpful, they ought to be receiving it." Krsek was convinced that it was harmless. He had taken it himself for a month to test it.

"I told them [Jacobson and Lippa]," said Krsek during a telephone interview in July 1987, "that if they would give me a large contract, I could supply the material for a third of the $250 a kilo I was charging them for material for clinical tests."

It was this remark that led to a contract between Houba and the PWA Health Group in New York City and subsequent sales to other PWA distribution groups throughout the country.

Despite the inconclusive results of the St. Luke's/Roosevelt clinical test, thousands of PWAs throughout the nation continued treatment with AL721. Although no figures are available (Lippa's estimate was 10,000), it is likely that at the end of 1987 the number of people taking AL721 approximated the number on AZT.

JACOBSON'S PEACE ENVOY

On November 27, 1987, the day after Thanksgiving Day, Robert Sturm, a young man in his late twenties hired by Jacobson a week earlier, met with a group of ACT UP and Lavender Hill Mob activists at Bill Bahlman's apartment in Greenwich Village. It was his mission to make peace with the AIDS activists and to promote sales of Ethigen's new over-the-counter "official" AL721.

Sturm had been thoroughly drilled to reply to the uncomfortable question, "Why did Ethigen wait so long to bring out AL721 as a food supplement?" The company had hoped to get FDA authorization quickly, he argued, so as to be able to sell it as a pharmaceutical. Insurance companies and Medicaid would then have paid for its distribution. If Ethigen had pursued the dual-track policy of selling AL721 as a food supplement while simultaneously pursuing FDA authorization as an ethical pharmaceutical, FDA would have denied Ethigen all possibility of drug approval. (Paradoxically, minutes later Sturm, too hastily prepared for his task, declared that Ethigen planned to continue FDA testing in an attempt at obtaining approval of AL721 as a pharmaceutical while simultaneously releasing it as a food supplement.)

According to Sturm, with authorization of distribution of AL721 for compassionate use in a major West European country, which he refused to name, market possibilities had changed, and Ethigen was able to approach major pharmaceutical houses to produce AL721. Upon being told that the country was known to be Britain, he assented with bewilderment. Sturm was asked to provide documentation on the British ruling. He promised to do so.

The documentation would never arrive.

With a newly established connection with Pfizer, Sturm declared, "Ethigen knows that they don't have to worry about having people out there wanting the product and not being able to get it." Ethigen had already done research, said Sturm, on the AL721 analogs being distributed by the various PWA health groups around the nation and found that none of these analogs was up to the standard "that both Ethigen and the community would like."

Tom Hannan, with whom Sturm met later that day, asked Sturm for documentation of this research. A week later Sturm telephoned to inform Tom that the research had been "informal," and no written documentation was available.

Another factor in Ethigen's decision to produce AL721 as a food supplement, according to Sturm, was FDA's reneging on a commitment to go directly from Phase I testing to Phase III. On the basis of that promise, Sturm declared, Ethigen had expected to be able to release AL721 as a pharmaceutical early in 1988.

(If AL721 had won approval "early" in 1988, it would have outraced even that FDA–NIH favorite, AZT!)

"A month or so ago," Sturm related, "FDA went back on its commitment and decided to require Phase II studies after all." Asked whether Ethigen could document FDA's change in policy, Sturm promised to request such documentation.

That documentation, too, would never arrive.

"I honestly believe," Sturm concluded, "or I would not be doing this job that [Ethigen's] intentions have always been appropriate. I interviewed Jake as much as he interviewed me. The only reason," said Sturm, "I can see for Jake being in this business really is because he wants the product out on the market. He doesn't need the money. I believe that he is in this business to try to get the best product out there at the best price he can."

Ethigen production of AL721, according to Sturm, was to commence in mid-December, and quantities would be available by mid-January.

That was not to be.

Hope, it seemed, sprang eternal at Ethigen, and in the third week in January 1988, Arnold Lippa, reduced from president of the company to a mere consultant, was announcing that a foreign firm had expressed interest in taking over Ethigen and installing a new management and "kicking Jacobson upstairs." The announcement proved abortive.

In February 1988 Linda Hunt reported that Ethigen had reached an arrangement with Abbott Laboratories and would be making AL721 available for general sale as a food supplement at the end of the month. Ethigen would spend no more money on clinical testing of AL721. "Why," she asked, "should we spend money to benefit all those who are distributing AL721 analogs?"

By the end of 1988 Ethigen had found two pharmacy outlets, one in New York City and the other in San Francisco. None of the PWA distribution groups ordered even a kilo from Ethigen. Early in 1989 Ethigen stock fell to $.05 from a high of almost $12 in June 1987.

HOUBA'S VICISSITUDES

The competition for the egg lecithin variant market was marked by vicious rumor-mongering by one of the West Coast distributors and by vindictiveness not only from Jacobson but, shamefully, from PWA activists in some of the distribution groups.

Thus one commercial distributor of an AL721 analog disseminated false rumors about the supposed inferior quality of competitors' products. One of the original PWA distributors of unauthorized therapies spread the rumor that the failure of other PWA groups in the nation to distribute the AL721 analog he favored was evidence of a "Jewish conspiracy." The head of a firm that distributed what he considered to be an inferior product, he pointed out, was Jewish and the manufacturer whose product this man imported was also Jewish. He could not be dissuaded of this canard even after being informed that the foreign manufacturer, in fact, was not Jewish at all. (On the other hand, the manufacturer whose product he himself touted was, unknown to him, Jewish.)

A far more serious problem arose from the rumor that none of the analogs being distributed in the United States resembled the original Israeli product. When the PWA Health Group submitted samples of the American Roland product to Skornik in May 1987, the Israeli physician noted that it differed in appearance and texture from the Israeli product (he made no intensive and comprehensive analysis of the American Roland product), but he advised the Health Group to go ahead with the distribution. Quoting only the first part of Skornik's statement, rumormongers telephoned PWAs to warn against the Health Group's material. They offered PWAs an analog supposedly identical to the Israeli product at $300 for a ten-day supply, and one PWA, intimidated by the warnings against the PWA Health Group product, persuaded his mother to mortgage her house in order to pay for the more expensive product. Fortunately, Joe Sonnabend, the man's physician, intervened in time to prevent this pointless action.

After Yehuda Skornik arranged with a South African concern for production of AL721 in South Africa, a nation that had not signed the international patent convention, "dissidents" in the United States announced that only the South African product was genuine and effective. They persuaded two Californians, one seriously ill with

AIDS, to empty their bank account to make a trip to South Africa for treatment. Upon arrival, the two discovered that they were the clinic's first patients. They were put up in a comfortable hotel. Over a period of two weeks they were given a series of clinical tests and treatment with the clinic's own AL721. "To prevent us from being bored," they reported, "we were taken on a safari, at no extra charge." When they returned home, they were given a small quantity of AL721 to tide them over. It was expected that they would continue to purchase their supplies from South Africa, at a price several times greater than that charged by the various PWA health groups.

Without asking his permission, the South African concern included Sonnabend's name on its letterhead as a member of the board of directors. Infuriated, Sonnabend demanded its removal. "We can provide those clinical tests right here," he declared. "People don't have to go to South Africa even though a safari can be very pleasant."

Passing through New York on his way to an international conference in Montreal, Dr. Barry Schub, the director of the National Institute for Virology in Johannesburg and head of the nation's AIDS research program, denied categorically any official connection with the South African clinic, a connection that the proponents of the South African clinic claimed to exist. He knew nothing about the clinic's operations. "It is purely a business enterprise," he declared.

Although the directors of Ethigen were disturbed generally by the proliferation of AL721 analogs, their anger was directed particularly at Krsek. Their representative Robert Sturm admitted that Ethigen found no fault with Houba's product, but he warned that Ethigen would take legal action if Houba continued "to violate" the AL721 patent. Indeed, a month after Sturm's visit to New York, on December 4, 1987, a Los Angeles law firm sent a letter to Houba headed "Infringement of Ethigen Patents" accusing Houba of violation of patent rights in "the distribution of significant quantities of Lipid compound to PWA Health Group of New York as well as the solicitation of additional orders from other groups throughout the United States." The letter demanded that he immediately desist in "the manufacture, use or sale of our client's patented Lipid products."

Houba's lawyers denied the allegations. Investigating the patent, Krsek and his lawyers had discovered that in developing AL721 in his laboratory at the Weizmann Institute, Shinitzky had combined pure PC, pure PE and pure neutral lipids in a 7:2:1 ratio. When Shinitzky attempted to repeat the 7:2:1 ratio in producing AL721 on a large scale, he obtained varying results. To meet patent office objections, he set a specification of 2 to 5 percent cholesterol; 2 to 5 percent phosphotidic acids; 15 to 35 percent PC; and from 40 to 80 percent neutral lipids—a far cry from strict 7:2:1 specifications. Indeed, the specifications were so broad that any manufacturer could produce an analog with impunity.

"The fact of the matter is," noted Krsek, "that most of the stuff out there [marketed in the United States] is almost a duplicate of Ethigen's by analysis though not made by Ethigen's method of extraction."

In any event, early in 1987 Krsek developed a new formula for his AL721 analog.

"We have cholesterol that's below two percent," he declared. "As for phosphotidic acid, we have less than one tenth of one percent. Our current product is, therefore, not the same as Ethigen's AL721, and Shinitzky is literally correct when he claims that Ethigen's is the only true 'AL721.' Our product is superior."

Krsek was also of the opinion that a ratio different from Shinitzky's 7:2:1 might be more effective. He did not want to become involved, however, in the testing required or in a conflict with the many groups that considered the 7:2:1 sacred.

In March 1988, four months after threatening Houba with a lawsuit, a contrite Jacobson sought a new contract with Houba to produce AL721 as a food supplement. Krsek did not exploit the opportunity to press for the $7,000 owed him by Ethigen. He yielded, too, when Jacobson said he could not meet Krsek's demand for cash payment. ("I'm a pussycat in such matters," he confessed.) Negotiations broke down, however, when Jacobson insisted upon production according to the original formula developed by Krsek; Krsek would only produce according to his new, improved formula—a formula over which Jacobson had no control.

Krsek and his associates spent weeks in testing their new analog formula before releasing it for shipment. An advance sample submitted to the New York PWA Health Group proved acceptable when tested; indeed, of all the analogs it most closely approached the 7:2:1 proportions. A quantity shipped to San Francisco, however, emitted a strong odor upon arrival. A sample of a subsequent New York shipment was rejected by the New York testing laboratory on the basis of an unacceptable level of isopropanol alcohol and significantly lower percentages of phospholipids than claimed.

Faced with alarm on the East and West coasts both because of the odor and the laboratory report, alarm intensified by Houba's most aggressive competitor, who telephoned around the country to warn that PWAs would be poisoned by the Houba product, Krsek recalled the shipments. He sent samples to laboratories in Chicago and St. Louis. Their analyses contradicted the New York laboratory's, showing the presence of only an infinitesimal amount of isopropanol alcohol and confirming the percentages of phospholipids claimed by Houba.

The unpleasant odor, Krsek discovered, resulted from an error by the packaging firm. During the filling process, egg oil spilled onto the rim of the cup. When the cup was sealed at a high temperature, the trapped egg oil was seared. Thus the obnoxious odor of burnt eggs. Krsek changed the method of packaging and further refined his product to reduce the alcohol content below a detectable amount.

Houba underwent other travails.

On October 31, 1987 Matt Galbraith, a staff writer for the local Indiana newspaper, the *South Bend Tribune*, reported that Houba was "involved in secret work on an 'AIDS vaccine.'" Utilizing the Freedom of Information Act, Galbraith obtained reports from the district office of FDA on Houba. Deletions in these reports roused his suspicions.

One day while waiting in line at a local bank, Krsek was warned that local citizens were talking about torching his plant because of their fear of the AIDS virus with which he was supposedly conducting experiments. On November 9, in a letter to Galbraith, Krsek emphatically denied that Houba was engaged in such research. He noted that "similar compositions to AL721 under the generic name of 'Lecithins' have been used in human foods for at least sixty years."

Although Galbraith published the substance of Krsek's reply, he continued his attack under the headline "AIDS drug lacks FDA approval." He reported the order from the Ethigen attorney to Houba to "cease and desist" in manufacturing and selling EL 1020, as the Houba product was called.

(How did the reporter obtain a copy of this letter?)

On March 2, 1988 Krsek received a regulatory letter from John P. Dempster, acting FDA district director, ordering Houba to desist from manufacture and distribution of the substance. Dempster charged that in an interview on an Indiana television station, Lin Zoller, one of Krsek's associates, had called the Houba product "a drug" and had made medical claims for it. Zoller denied the charge, and when Krsek requested a transcript of the interview, the station refused to provide it.

The threat to all AL721 analogs was clear, and leaders in the AIDS community sought clarification from the national office of FDA. The *New York Native* published an article calling the case to the attention of the gay community and quoting Michael Callen of the New York PWA Health Group as saying, "It would be a devastating blow if FDA decides to shut Houba down." Callen called Houba "responsible and reliable in its supply" of its AL721 analog.

On March 27, 1988 the *South Bend Tribune* announced: "Changes by Houba avert FDA charges." Dempster had expressed satisfaction with Houba's decision to change the name of its product from EL 1020 to Houba Egg Lecithin and to add a clear designation as a food supplement. (In fact, EL 1020 had been clearly identified as a food supplement.) During this fracas, the rumor spread, encouraged by Houba's rumormongering competitor, that Houba had been shut down by FDA.

Again in September 1988 FDA investigated Houba. It charged that lots of a new syrup egg lecithin developed by Houba contained substances not in conformity with food labeling regulations. Houba recalled all lots and discontinued the production of the syrup product. It continued selling its original "butter" product.

By January 1989 Houba had developed a new capsule product, easy to ship and convenient for clients to use. Having obtained advance FDA approval for this new product, Houba was preparing to market the capsules in February.

In selecting among the numerous AL721 analogs, however, distribution groups around the country, and often their medical consultants as well, were hampered by a lack of scientific sophistication in regard to the production and testing of the analogs. When Blum of American Roland tested an Ethigen product at Tom Hannan's request (he was unaware that it had been manufactured by Houba), Tom, misreading the printout of the results, announced that the Houba product was not up to par and that the clinical test held at St. Luke's/Roosevelt Hospital might, therefore, have reached inconclusive results. Months later, informed of Hannan's interpretation of his analysis of the Houba product, an indignant Mel Blum insisted that his test demonstrated that the Houba product was of comparable quality to American Roland's and to Shinitzky's.

It was because of the bewilderment among PWA groups as to which product to promote and because of the potential danger in errors like Tom's that I asked Blum and Krsek, industrial competitors but competent scientists, to draft criteria for evaluating AL721 analogs. Without mention of his name, Tom's misreading of Blum's testing of a Houba product was offered as one of the reasons for the development of this report. The leaders of the PWA Health Group adjudged inclusion of this incident an affront and reacted with vindictiveness against Houba and against the compiler of the report.[2]

Perhaps at the instigation of one or more of Houba's competitors, FDA renewed its attack on Houba. Krsek was compelled once again to recall large shipments of his product and became, as a result, heavily indebted to both the New York and the San Francisco distribution groups. Upon the resolution once again of his problem with FDA, the two groups refused to accept payment of the Houba debt in deliveries of the revised and approved product or to place new orders until he had paid his debt. When the New York group brought suit against Houba for the money owed, Krsek paid the debt out of his own pocket in order to save his firm from bankruptcy.

Discouraged by FDA persecution and by the vindictiveness of the New York and San Francisco groups, Krsek abandoned production of the AL721 analog although he was still obtaining orders amounting to about $10,000 a month from other groups. What had started as a generous effort to assist the PWAs ended in general ill will and a Pyrrhic victory for rancorous activists.[3]

With the development of new therapies and refinement in the administration of AZT, AL721 ceased to be a major therapy among PWAs although sales of the egg lecithin variant continued, if in decreasing quantities.

Dr. Bernard Bihari of Downstate Medical College, the initial experimenter with AL721, continues to promote its use. At a panel discussion on January 19, 1988 he noted that in the limited studies at St. Luke's/Roosevelt and in Israel, "reverse transcriptase [an enzyme produced by HIV] was reduced by 90 percent. None of the toxic anti-virals," he declared, "reduce reverse transcriptase this much. AL721 fits the criteria [for alternative therapies] . . . : it is non-toxic and there is a scientific basis for it."

---

[2] Upon being asked by a publisher to offer a judgment of the manuscript of this book, one of the leaders of the PWA Health Group dismissed it in a few abrupt sentences as unworthy of publication. In December 1990 Tom gave assurance that he was not the writer of this evaluation.

[3] Stephen Levine's company, a distributor but not a manufacturer of an AL721 analog, was also threatened by FDA. Jay Lipner, an AIDS community member of the AIDS Roundtable of the Institute of Medicine, interceded with FDA and quashed the projected action.

In an editorial in the December 12, 1988 issue of the *GMHC Treatment Issues* entitled "Is It Time to Retire AL721?" however, Barry Gingell, who had used AL721 with positive though limited effect, summed up what had become a general view in the United States. Until recently, he wrote, "it just didn't seem that enough clinical data had been accumulated, and very little was published to venture some kind of opinion about the drug. . . . Two unimpressive studies," he noted, "were presented at the Stockholm AIDS conference which did not show convincing improvement in people taking the drug." With the eight patients enrolled in the St. Luke's/Roosevelt study, "there were no significant improvements in T-cell numbers or of p24 antigen levels . . . . 4 out of the 8 patients have progressed to AIDS over the subsequent 14 months. The number of patients on AL721 followed by local physicians," he noted, "total much more than the St. Luke's study. When asked whether they felt that AL721 had any positive clinical effect on patients, physicians consistently answer 'No.' "

◆ ◆ ◆

In the fall of 1987 Michael May, the individual who had initiated the worldwide publicity on AL721, returned to work as a choral conductor, and a concert at Carnegie Hall served as a celebration of the recovery of his strength. Although the next month he suffered an intense emotional shock with the death of his lover from AIDS, May steeled himself and undertook one engagement after another as a conductor. Maintaining a religious faith in AL721, he rejected Skornik's advice not to rely solely on AL721 as a therapy. After his decline became impossible to deny, at any momentary renewal of energy he insisted that his recovery was once again on track. He even volunteered to serve as a "buddy" to another PWA, not as ill as he but lacking his morale. Ironically, at the request of his chorus, despite his own misgivings, he conducted the Mozart Requiem. It proved to be his own requiem. He came down with severe and unremitting diarrhea. In the hospital, Madeline, one of his choristers, took turns with his mother in changing his bedclothes. When his mother urged him to fight on, he replied, "Do you want me to continue to suffer?"

On June 30, 1988 Michael May died.

◆ ◆ ◆

After repeated and abortive announcements of imminent rescue by new investors, American and foreign, by December 1989, at the expiration of the Israeli license, Jacobson sought an extension for a last-minute effort. In February 1990 the license reverted to the Israelis. Several months later Jacobson moved to Hong Kong.

Much of the rumor circulated about Ethigen, according to Arnold Lippa, was mere melodramatic fantasy. The company had confronted difficult objective problems. It had required years to develop mass production of AL721 that matched the small and easily controlled quantities produced in Shinitzky's laboratory at the

Weizmann Institute and to learn how to store and preserve large quantities of the compound. Even Krsek's product, developed under Shinitzky's supervision, Lippa declared, was uneven and Houba shipments sometimes had to be returned for re-formulation. Fulton Crews of the University of Florida at Gainesville, a leading researcher in AL721 and a signer of the 1985 *New England Journal of Medicine* article, had tested analogs sold by the PWA distribution groups and found them unsatisfactory. (After a similar investigation, Mel Blum of American Roland dismissed several of these products as of "mere cosmetic [manufacturing] quality.") According to Lippa, a precise 7:2:1 ratio (achievable in Shinitzky's laboratory) was essential for effectiveness, a ratio rarely attained or maintained in mass production. The difficulty in producing sufficient quantities of first-quality AL721, declared Lippa, hampered the development of clinical trials. As for the uncertain results in the St. Luke's/Roosevelt test, Lippa noted that during the extension of the test the researchers eliminated the requirement that AL721 be taken on an empty stomach or at least after a nonfat meal, a requirement upon which Shinitzky had insisted.

In the summer of 1987 Lippa sought FDA authorization of a multicenter test of AL721 with individuals in an advanced state of HIV infection. To avoid endangerment of life-threatened subjects through the use of placebos, he proposed using AZT, the single drug approved by FDA as an AIDS therapy, as the control in a decisive test of the efficacy of AL721. When FDA failed to reply to this application for an unprecedented comparison of AZT, the "official" drug, with another therapeutic compound, Ethigen was unable to raise funds in a stock offering in 1988, and the demise of the company became inevitable.

FDA, according to Lippa, in an unprecedented action transferred the administration of clinical testing of AL721 from Ethigen to the administrators of the ATEU program. FDA also insisted upon a dosage-ranging test, which Lippa insisted was not necessary after the St. Luke's/Roosevelt clinical test and the tests conducted by the Israelis.

AL721 had never received, Lippa insists, the large-scale testing it deserves. The Israelis, he notes, were at the end of 1990 still using it with some one hundred individuals with HIV infection.

PART II

CHAPTER

Mr. Reagan Appoints
a Commission

With the appointment in the summer of 1987 of a Presidential Commission on the Human Immunodeficiency Virus Epidemic mandated to evolve a national policy on the epidemic, the AIDS struggle entered a new phase. AIDS activists could claim major credit in forcing an apathetic and uncompassionate president to at least make a pretense at fulfilling his obligations as commander-in-chief in what had evolved into a grave national war. Reviving militancy in a demoralized gay community, in street demonstrations and with varied imaginative pressure tactics, these activists exposed the ramifications of the crisis to the Congress and the American people. They gained sophistication in political maneuvering and insights into the workings of agencies entrusted with research and clinical testing. They abandoned illusions about the relationship between pharmaceutical giants and FDA and NIH. Assuming responsibilities proper to government agencies, AIDS organizations were publicizing promising new drugs, organizing distributions of unauthorized therapies and even developing community research projects.

Thus the events in previous chapters represent a prelude to a new phase of the "winter war," a phase in which activists like Martin Delaney, Bill Bahlmann, Tom Hannan, Barry Gingell, Iris Long and Michael Callen along with many others made decisive contributions to the deliberations of the new commission and pressured it to engage in bold probings of fundamental questions exposed by the AIDS crisis.

◆ ◆ ◆

In November 1983, two years after the definition of the AIDS disease, in a report entitled "The Federal Response to AIDS," the House Committee on Government

Operations recommended the convening of "a panel of appropriate professionals . . . to facilitate the coordination and farsighted planning of our national response to AIDS." After another four years of administration inertia, in a report entitled "AIDS Prevention: Views on the Administration's [1988] Budget Proposals," prepared for a subcommittee of the Senate Committee on Appropriations, the General Accounting Office quoted health service experts and state and local health department officials as recommending "a full-scale federally coordinated campaign against AIDS" and as complaining "that the perceived lack of federal leadership is at least as troublesome as estimated shortfalls in the budget."

On May 4, 1987 (the very day the PWA Health Group in New York held its first distribution of an AL721 analog), seven years after the identification of the disease Ronald Reagan announced his intention to create a Presidential Commission on the Human Immunodeficiency Virus Epidemic with a mandate to formulate a national strategy for combating the epidemic.

People throughout the country responded to the president's announcement with misgivings. Few if any of those involved in combating the AIDS epidemic had confidence that the Reagan administration, lacking in compassion for those suffering and dying in the scourge and oblivious to the threat the epidemic represented to the security of the nation, was seriously determined to evolve and effect an aggressive national AIDS policy.

On June 24 Reagan appointed Dr. W. Eugene Mayberry, the chief executive officer of the Mayo Clinic, as chairman of a commission that would advise him and relevant officials "on the public health dangers, including the medical, legal, ethical, social and economic impact, from the spread of the HIV and resulting illnesses."

"AIDS," admitted Mayberry, "is not my field of expertise."

With a budget of between $900,000 and $1.5 million, the new Commission was to draft recommendations on research, treatment, ethics and international collaboration. It was to hold its first meeting in September and to issue a report in June 1988.

Leaders of the AIDS community as well as other public opinion makers expressed outrage at both the lack of qualifications and biases of most of the appointees, who almost without exception favored mandatory testing for the AIDS virus, a measure opposed by an overwhelming majority of public health officials and by the National Academy of Sciences Panel on AIDS as raising "serious problems of ethics and feasibility."

Although the epidemic raged with disproportionate virulence among minorities, only one black and no Hispanics were among the appointees. Against the opposition of Gary Bauer, the presidential domestic policy adviser, a single member of the gay community was appointed—Frank Lilly, chairman of the Genetics Department at the Albert Einstein Medical Center in New York City and formerly a board member of the Gay Men's Health Crisis. "The president was well-advised to put a gay on this commission," Lilly declared. "There would have been a terrible hullabaloo from the main people influenced by this disease if he had not."

To the charge of partisan bias on the Commission, Bauer retorted: "Were we to appoint people hostile to the president? Were we to appoint supporters of Ted Kennedy? . . . When we have seats to fill, we'll fill some of them with our friends." Colleen Conway-Welch, dean of the School of Nursing at Vanderbilt University and wife of a key fundraiser in Vice President George Bush's presidential campaign, declared: "I don't think being married to a Republican fund-raiser was the reason I was chosen, but it probably didn't hurt."

The rationales for the other appointments were more tenuous:

- Dr. Theresa Crenshaw, appointed because of her experience in sex education, had sought to exclude students with HIV infection from the San Diego public schools and scoffed at the promotion of the use of condoms in AIDS prevention education. In contradiction to all reputable scientific opinion, she had declared that "AIDS could be transmitted through mosquitoes, household pets, food handlers or public toilets, and infected children should be barred from school."

After appearing with Dr. Crenshaw on a talk show, Dr. Donald I. Abrams of San Francisco General Hospital exclaimed: "I couldn't believe this woman is really a physician. I felt she was dangerously misinformed."

- Penny Pullen, a member of the Illinois legislature and sponsor of mandatory testing legislation and an associate of Phyllis Schafly in opposing ratification of the Equal Rights Amendment, considered AIDS as divine punishment for sexual deviation.
- John J. Creedon, president of the Metropolitan Life Insurance Company, was an advocate of blood testing in screening applicants for insurance.
- Cory Servass, editor and publisher of the *Saturday Evening Post*, in 1986 claimed that she had discovered a "cure" for AIDS based on health foods, vitamins and an antiviral drug used for herpes; she presented "medical minute" health tips on various television programs, including the Rev. Pat Robertson's fundamentalist hour. Her husband was Indiana chairman of the Pat Robertson for President campaign.
- Richard M. DeVos, president of the Amway Corporation, whose only qualification seemed to be that he was the largest single contributor to Reagan's 1980 presidential campaign as well as a member of the board of the Robert Schuller Ministries, a fundamentalist religious organization.
- John Cardinal O'Connor, the archbishop of New York, had a reputation as one of the most homophobic of the American Roman Catholic bishops.
- Admiral (ret.) James D. Watkins was a former chief of naval operations.

Regarding the composition of the Commission, Dr. Mervyn Silverman, president of the American Foundation for AIDS Research, declared: "I'm underwhelmed." The response of David G. Ostrow, a member of the AIDS Expert Advisory Panel of the American Medical Association, was more comprehensive. "The absence from the commission," he said, "of anyone experienced in the treatment of people with AIDS and of AIDS researchers or public health experts should be a warning to the medical profession of the direction U.S. AIDS policy is taking."

Even within the Reagan administration there were discordant reactions. Martin Delaney reported that "a highlight of the meeting [he attended with FDA Commissioner Frank Young and a number of Young's colleagues in July] came with a mention of the newly appointed president's commission. The groans and raucous laughter convinced me," Delaney reported, "that I and the others in the room were not entirely on opposite sides." In October in a conversation with Delaney, C. Boyden Gray, a Bush aide, scoffed, "That commission is going to take a year and a half just to figure out what the questions are."

The Commission immediately confronted problems. The chairman was unable to fill more than three of fifteen staff positions. After the first Commission hearings on September 10, the *Chicago Tribune* reported that panel members expressed alarm at what they called "a credibility gap" between federal efforts to find a cure for the fatal affliction and a widespread public perception that little was being done. "We have a war of words almost more than a war on AIDS," the paper quoted Commission member DeVos as saying. "Why is it with all this expertise and knowledge—why is it the American people aren't buying [government explanations]?" William B. Walsh asked, "If everyone [in government] is doing what they say they're doing, I don't understand why anyone is sick. What seems to be lacking is a national strategy." Commenting on Walsh's remark, Ralph Bledsoe, executive secretary of the White House Domestic Policy Council, quipped: "Welcome to the federal government."

At the first hearings of the Commission, ACT UP staged a major demonstration with posters calling the Commission "the Mickey Mouse Club" and showing Donald Duck with the caption "Ron, you forgot to include me on your Commission."

On September 8 counsel representing a group of six New York and Washington, D.C., organizations—the National Association of People with AIDS, the PWA Coalition, the GMHC, the National Minority AIDS Council, the Public Citizen Health Research Group and the American Public Health Association along with Michael Callen as an individual complainant—delivered a letter to the president and to the secretary of Health and Human Services requesting that they "take actions to rectify the imbalance on the Commission" by appointing "additional members . . . to represent the excluded views and interests." The plaintiffs offered to recommend "qualified individuals who could represent the excluded interests."

On October 1 Linda Sheaffer, selected as Commission executive director upon the recommendation of Secretary Otis Bowen of HHS, was compelled to resign. (At the time of her appointment Ms. Sheaffer, who had no professional background in AIDS, gave assurance that she had been "an avid reader about the issue.") Sheaffer declared in a two-sentence statement to the press that the chairman asked her to resign "because of internal disagreements within the commission that had nothing to do with my overall performance as the executive director."

On October 7 the counsel for the complainant AIDS organizations received a letter from the counsel to the president denying the request for a change in the composition of the Commission "on the ground that the Commission is currently balanced because it has among its members the head of the Mayo Clinic, the Indiana Health Commissioner, who is Black, individuals of both sexes, and a member of the gay community."

That very day Commission Chairman Mayberry and Vice Chairman Woodrow A. Myers, the Indiana health commissioner and the single black on the Commission, both resigned. Mayberry issued no statement, but Myers declared there was "not complete support of Dr. Mayberry's position nor of [his own] role as vice chairman" and that they "did not receive a full degree of support from the administration."

On October 11, under the headline "The Reagan AIDS Strategy in Ruins," the *New York Times* proclaimed editorially: "While the AIDS epidemic gets its grip on America, Mr. Reagan's Administration spouts, postures and neglects effective measures to curb it. The President's commission on AIDS has begun to self-destruct." Of retired Admiral James D. Watkins, the president's new appointee as chairman, the *Times* commented: "He is an able leader but knows even less about AIDS than his fellow commissioners. To expect this motley group to develop a competent strategy is like asking a panel of physicians to design the navy's next attack submarine."

On October 14, 1987 the six complainant organizations filed a civil action in the United States District Court in the District of Columbia against the president, the secretary of Health and Human Services and the Presidential Commission. The suit charged that the members of the Commission did "not represent the interests of people with AIDS, or those who provide services, such as health care and counseling, to people with AIDS, or of the communities that have been hardest hit by the disease"; that most had "little or no experience with or expertise on AIDS issues"; that four people on the Commission had "publicly advanced positions that run counter to the interests of those directly affected by AIDS and that conflict with the mainstream views held by the vast majority of those with experience or expertise on AIDS issues" and that "the Commission include[d] no representatives of those who hold countervailing views, including individuals with expertise and experience on AIDS." The plaintiffs asked the court "to preliminarily enjoin the AIDS Commission from proceeding with its work unless and until it contains balanced membership in accordance with the requirements of FACA" (the Federal Advisory Committee Act).

◆ ◆ ◆

Implicit in the criticism of the composition of the Presidential Commission was more than a belated outcry at Reagan's lack of compassion and denigration of the gravity of the epidemic. The angry outcry represented, in addition, a belated welling that year of repugnance at the values and goals of Reaganism in general.

Indeed, if presidential neglect in the AIDS crisis was beyond "excuse," it was not beyond "comprehension." Soon after his election as president, Reagan announced: "What I want to see above all is that this country remain a country where someone can always get rich." Five years later at the 1986 graduation exercises of the University of California School of Business Administration, to enthusiastic applause and laughter, Wall Street arbitrageur Ivan Boesky wittily summed up Reaganite Americanism, declaring: "Greed is all right. . . . Greed is healthy. You can be greedy and still feel good about yourself."

The 1987 edition of "The Forbes Four Hundred: The Richest People in America" confirmed the achievement of Reagan's goal, reporting that from 1982 to 1987 the average net worth of the "400" rose from $230 to $550 million; and the minimum net worth, from $91 to $225 million. The combined wealth of the 400 almost quadrupled, rising from $64 to $220 billion. The number of billionaires in the United States almost doubled from 1986 to 1987, from twenty-six to forty-nine (up from thirteen in 1982), a statistic that could hardly be approached in any other country in the world.

But greed was accompanied by more than "feeling good."

In May 1987, after noting that the "clarion call" of the Reagan administration had been "Enrich thyself," *Time* magazine pointed out that this administration "from its very beginning has been riddled from top to bottom with allegations of impropriety and corruption. More than 100 members," the magazine declared, "have had ethical or legal charges leveled against them. The number is without precedent. This can hardly be what the administration means when it talks about 'traditional values.'"

Official policy and action in regard to AIDS would hardly be immune from this pervasive corruption.

At the time of the appointment of the Presidential Commission, a clash over national values and priorities was beginning to emerge. "Total fund requests for the 'Star Wars' Strategic Defense Initiative, $5 billion," observed the Friends Committee on National Legislation, "are more than the combined totals requested for the women, infants and children's nutrition program, low-income-home-energy assistance, Native American health and education, community service block grants and the Legal Services Corporation. The $80 million requested for the emergency food and shelter program for the homeless is less than the request for four air-cushion landing crafts at $21.3 million each."

"Enrich thyself" ideals also brought a cost in the tone of national life. On February 7, 1988 *New York Times* architecture editor Paul Goldberger remarked on a simultaneous publication of an opinion survey that revealed that becoming wealthy was more important to college freshmen than developing a "meaningful philosophy of life" and the appearance on the best-seller list of *The Art of the Deal* by Forbes "400" billionaire entrepreneur Donald Trump. "Mr. Trump's considerable riches," commented Goldberger, "are his business, not ours. The eminence he enjoys today, however, is something that our society has conferred upon him. It is our way of telling him how well he has embodied our values, how much he represents what, deep down, so many of us want to be. If the reports of the values of today's college freshmen are correct, Mr. Trump will retain his stature for a long time."

At a Brooklyn, New York, conference on "AIDS in the Black Population," on

October 15, 1987, the very day that Admiral Watkins assumed the chairmanship of the Presidential Commission, Dr. Reed Tuckson, D.C. Commissioner of Public Health and chairman of the Committee on Medical Legislation of the National Medical Association, proclaimed:

> AIDS presents a major threat to the civilization of America. How we come together and face the multiple challenges presented by this disease will define the character of our society. Our values, principles, ethics and morality are central to this fight. Equally important are our competence and compassion. . . . It is how we come together as a civilized people that will determine the success of this country in waging the war against AIDS.

As Dr. Tuckson so eloquently proclaimed, the AIDS epidemic was a testing of the nation—a testing at a time when the nation was being guided by a "summer soldier and sunshine patriot, hardly a winter soldier."

The Admiral Pulls a Surprise

On October 16, 1987, upon assuming his post as Commission chairman, Admiral Watkins responded to the widespread ridicule and cynicism being expressed regarding the commission: "While the Commission has received a great deal of adverse publicity because of its shaky and controversial start, I want you to know today that I with the support of my colleagues on the Commission intend to pull things together and to move forward aggressively."

Two months later, on December 16, the District Court judge denied the complaint in the class action suit seeking redress in the composition of the Presidential Commission. An amended complaint filed on January 12, 1988, also proved abortive, but by this time the AIDS community, the media and the public at large were reconsidering their initial derogation of the Commission. A *New York Times* editorial on February 28 summed up a general turnabout in attitude:

> Last October, when Admiral Watkins became the new chairman, it seemed inconceivable that the President's ignorant, bickering AIDS commission could be constructive. "The White House has no AIDS strategy and a commission with no chance of producing one," this paper said. Admiral Watkins has now confounded such criticism. He has blunted the far-out ideas of some fellow panelists and the Administration's urge to make widespread testing the chief weapon against AIDS. He has perceived the need for quicker development and FDA approval of drugs to help those already infected.
>
> In five months, Admiral Watkins has learned what the Administration failed to grasp in five years. The urgent need is to stop crying wolf about tertiary transmission and to deal instantly with transmission among drug addicts, the wolf that is at the door.

What caused this reversal in judgment? Was the original harsh dismissal of the Commission by the media and the AIDS community hasty and unfounded?

Interviewed on April 12, 1988, Tom Brandt, the Commission's coordinator for communications, noted that upon his appointment, the original chairman, W. Eugene Mayberry, a physician with no experience with Washington politics, had been assured that he would be able to function on a part-time basis as Commission chairman while carrying on his responsibilities at the Mayo Clinic. (This assurance of a "part-time" assignment exposed the half-hearted support the administration would provide to the Commission's mission!) On the other hand, the Commission was given a broad mandate, too broad for a part-time chairman. Furthermore, according to Brandt, any Federal AIDS commission, "was bound to be controversial . . . and you were going to be ragged on from right and left. The intensity of the attacks probably caught Mayberry and some of the others by surprise."

With the intense interest of the public in a commission appointed so belatedly in the epidemic, Brandt declared, the media began interviewing members before the Commission had even held an organizational meeting. Fundamental organizational questions had not been addressed: how often the Commission would meet, whom it would consult, in what order issues would be investigated, what the parameters of its efforts were to be, and so forth. In addition, no staff had been hired. Thus the impression of disorganization, incompetence and discord.

Walking in the door as the new chairman in mid-October, Brandt recalled, Admiral Watkins found two staff people overwhelmed by the ringing of the telephones. A backlog of unanswered mail was piled on desks. Applying the organizational experience and leadership abilities of a former Chief of Naval Operations, Watkins appointed a new executive director, Polly L. Gault, and with her assistance assembled a "top-level" staff. (Polly had been on the Hill for about six years serving as staff director of a Senate subcommittee overseeing about $25 billion of public health funds.)

In an interview in March 1988, six months after Admiral Watkins assumed the chairmanship, Frank Hagan, the Commission's media consultant, rejected the initial assertions by the media and the AIDS community that Commission members were political appointees ill-equipped for their task. Frank Lilly with thirty years of work with retroviruses and Burton Lee, a lymphoma expert with considerable experience with patients with HIV infection, Hagan insisted, were well-equipped to participate in the Commission's investigations. He noted that the New York Roman Catholic archdiocese under the leadership of John Cardinal O'Connor operated some of the finest AIDS facilities in the city and that Colleen Conway-Welch, dean of the School of Nursing at Vanderbilt University, had expertise in a fundamental area of the Commission's responsibilities.

Hagan complained of gross media distortion in early reportage on the Commission. He recalled watching with misgivings as Theresa Crenshaw, a Commission member who had been roundly attacked for outspoken prejudice against people with AIDS, appeared at a press interview. "After what I had heard and read about her," Hagan reported, "I said to myself, 'Thank God, she didn't say anything that could be considered controversial.' Then I read the interview, and it was the most distorted article I had ever seen in print. Thereafter, instead of calling her Dr. Crenshaw, I called her 'Miss Quote.'" On another occasion, a Washington reporter quoted her as expressing anger because the Commission refused to send her to Sweden to meet someone who claimed he became infected with HIV merely by shaking hands. "At the time this interview was supposedly taking place," said Hagan, "I was with her at the Mother Teresa Hospice in New York, where she massaged the back of a PWA who was very thin and was complaining that his bones ached. When she went to smear him with an ointment without putting on a rubber glove, he said 'No, no, don't do that.' She said, 'You can't get AIDS by touching someone.' 'No, no,' the patient insisted, 'the ointment smells like shit, put the glove on so that you won't stink.' She laughed. While I was watching this, some crazy reporter was recounting that an interview was taking place at that very moment in another city."

Cory Servass, publisher of the *Saturday Evening Post*, like Crenshaw, was a particular target of criticism of the media and of the AIDS community. A product of middle-class, Bible-belt America, according to Hagan, she had been fed information by people who had a very particular point of view, and she expressed this point of view very positively. "Now she's meeting people," Hagan declared, "and she's hearing their stories and understanding their frustrations. . . . Now Servass, Martin Delaney [of Project Inform] and I agree on three quarters of the pie. Last year we would have thrown the pie at her."

Hagan's reaction to Cardinal O'Connor was more complex. Raised and educated as a Catholic, Hagan left the church, disillusioned by its attitude toward gays and lesbians. He speaks of "a Catholic church with 18th century values, 19th century application and 20th century problems." He felt particular resentment at the Cardinal because of the Cardinal's open hostility to gays and lesbians. "The Cardinal," he says, "knew I was one of 'them' and expected me to dislike him."

An experience during a visit with Theresa Crenshaw to St. Clare's Hospital caused Frank to modify his suspicions of the prelate. Patients in the AIDS ward were engaged in a Halloween room-decorating contest that was to be judged by the Cardinal. "I want to make sure that you vote for my room in the voting box at the end of the hall," exclaimed a patient in a room decorated with toilet paper streamers and get-well cards. "The Card and I are real close," he declared. "He comes around and talks to everybody. He doesn't push the Catholic business down your throat."

One day Hagan found himself in the Cardinal's company on their way to a reception. "I know you know that I don't agree with everything you stand for," Hagan said to the Cardinal, "but you're a Commission member, and you're dealing with the gay community. If there is any way that I can help you, I'll be glad to do so." The Cardinal responded with a look "somewhere between shock and amazement." "If, indeed, I need help, I will ask you," he said, "and thank you for the offer."

(Hagan was operating in a particular relationship with the Cardinal. His favorable remarks about the prelate, remarks offering insight into the complexity of the Cardinal's stance toward the epidemic, were not shared by AIDS activists. Angered by his dogmatic and uncompromising public denunciations of homosexuality, stubborn opposition to education on safe sex and the use of condoms, they conducted repeated protest demonstrations at St. Patrick's Cathedral and attacked him as a more negative than positive force in the AIDS struggle.)

If they had investigated the Admiral's background, the media and the AIDS community would not have been confounded by the turnaround he achieved within the Commission.

According to Admiral Watkins, Bob Tuttle, the personnel director at the White House, called him one day to say that the White House wanted a military man on the panel. Watkins's name, Tuttle declared, had been proposed because of his background in personnel work and because of his four-year experience with the president, from 1982 to 1986, as Chief of Naval Operations. The White House knew that, in general, he was "in their camp." Watkins asked how much time he would have to devote to the assignment and was told "a day and a half a month." He replied, "I know that's not true, but if it's three days a month, OK, I'll do it."

In a February 28, 1989 interview for a PBS television program entitled "The Education of Admiral Watkins," the Admiral claimed that he had not understood why he had been selected for the Commission: "I've always been healthy, my kids were healthy. Health has never been an issue for my family. I've always considered my annual physical examinations demeaning. . . . Why put me on?"

In fact, the Admiral was not so unsophisticated or devoid of experience. During the equal opportunity upheaval in the early 1970s, Watkins was appointed by Admiral Hyman Zumwalt, his mentor in the service, to be the Navy's first director for enlisted personnel. Subsequently, in the latter part of the decade during the difficult transition from the draft to the all-volunteer military, he was promoted to the post of Chief of Naval Personnel. Involved in the disadvantaged youth receiving project set up for the "100,000 kids to whom the judge would say, 'If you go to the Navy, we won't send you to prison for this felony,'" Watkins developed alcohol prevention and rehabilitation programs. "We got into drug testing," he recounted,

> organized a family service center and set up child day care centers. I saw lots of young kids unready for the work force, unhealthy and poorly motivated, with a low average reading level. Ninety percent had high school diplomas, particularly among the minorities, who had been pushed out of school with a diploma with an F or a D average, without counseling and with no hope of survival out in the private sector. Many were rejected by the Navy because we couldn't remediate them to above a sixth-grade reading level. I became involved in the human side of the problem, and it became my life, fighting for these people on Capitol Hill as a kind of union leader, demanding programs that we needed in order to survive, all the social support networks that had to be built under the all-volunteer military concept.

In 1985 Watkins was informed that the Navy was going to be the first service to employ the new test for sero-positivity, beginning with about 4,500 sailors on board the U.S.S. Midway. Homeported in Japan, many in the Midway crew were married to Japanese. "We had no guidance," recalled Admiral Watkins. "We had to build our own policy. There were difficult decisions. What if you have a married man with children and family who is found seropositive? What if you find a sailor married to a Japanese national? Are you going to shoot him? Bring him home? Put him before a courtmartial?"

Watkins set the policy that a sero-positive person would be sent home to a regional medical center, where he would remain actively employed. "Even at that time," he recalled, "we knew from the Surgeon-General that there was no evidence of casual transmission. We showed sensitivity to the people, maintaining as much confidentiality as possible. The individual gets absorbed in a major regional area like San Diego, Norfolk or Pensacola. Only his superior officer knows of his condition."

What differences would the Admiral have made in the composition of the Commission if he had had a role in the appointments?

> I would have asked, what do we want to achieve? You [the president] have asked us ethics, you've asked us financial, you have asked us social questions. I would have wanted a public health person. I would have wanted a black. I would have wanted a Hispanic. I would have picked somebody in the financial world who really understood cost–benefit analysis, cost management, in touch with health service, who understood Medicare, Medicaid, the complexities of the health care financing system, somebody highly respected. I would probably have wanted somebody that's really been into social work . . . that has had their hands dirtied in the real world in providing help to others.

A person with AIDS?

"I think I would have, but a person that is going to have the strength and depth and is going to be a real help, not just because he has AIDS. Now that could well have been the gay member. . . . That would have been very helpful."

How did Admiral Watkins overcome these perceived lacks?

> I augmented the staff with the kinds of background that we didn't have on the commission. Polly [Gault, the Commission's executive director] and I sat down and said, "Let's get a person with AIDS." . . . The friend of one of our staff people who came to us from the White House . . . she happens to be American Indian . . . knew Philip [a PWA]. We brought Philip right in. He can't do a lot of things [because of his uncertain health], but he can do a lot of things we have to have done, and he felt good about it. We brought him in and we listened to him. And we heard a story of discrimination that is typical, right here in D.C. . . . Most of the Commission heard his story. I brought in two Hispanics, one of them a lawyer. . . . We bounce off ideas on Jane Delgado, a close friend of Polly's, all the time. She's happily a member of the Leadership Coalition on AIDS, where she represents the Hispanic community. . . . We had blacks, including Jackie Knox, a wonderful person from the Hill. We have a couple of gays on the staff. They work out of New York and were able to ensure that we had representation among our witnesses from the gay communities. . . . We wanted to hear from everybody. We had a nice cross section within the staff that

helped counterbalance either the perception or the reality of inadequacies in the backgrounds of the Commissioners.

Why did the Admiral not publicize his effort to compensate for a lack of balance among the commissioners through the appointment of a well-balanced staff?

"We had an ACLU suit against us [ACLU et al., seeking expansion in the membership of the Commission to achieve representation of minorities and of the AIDS community]. We couldn't talk about it."

Regarding the criticism that the Commission membership was not representative, Commissioner Burton Lee III of Memorial Sloan Kettering Medical Center in New York, noted:

> You can't have thirteen people on a Commission and not have 20 million people call to complain that they weren't represented. . . . My first reaction to the make-up of the Commission was pleasure that it was not just a medical commission, which would have been mired in a lot of medical detail better dealt with elsewhere. We had a broader based group that would be looking for policy and priorities in dealing with the AIDS problem along with a big spectrum of activities—legal, financial, social and international. When Myers and Mayberry resigned, we did work hard for the appointments of Beny Primm as a drug addiction expert and a representative of the black community and of Kristine M. Gebbie, an excellent public health person. We also secured appointment of Admiral Watkins as chairman. But I never expected that all thirteen people would be just who I might want. . . . The people that I would have expected to be the most hard-core, business-oriented, bottom-line, have been among our most sympathetic and concerned individuals on the Commission about the personal problems related to AIDS.

Conway-Welch had the impression "that certain of the Commissioners came to the Commission with certain concerns, and they have explored these concerns and learned more about them, and their attitudes have changed. We have all developed a keener appreciation of each other's point of view. It was one of the strong points of the Commission that we were a kind of grassroots with varied backgrounds, varied attitudes and value systems."

The Crisis Confronting the Commission

"Turning the Commission around" meant rendering it accessible to new ideas and mobilizing it to evolve a national program for dealing with an epidemic the gravity of which was scarcely appreciated initially by the Commission members.

On September 1, 1987, a week before the Commission began its operations, FDA Commissioner Frank Young warned at an Institute of Medicine conference that AIDS had "the potential to be the most devastating infectious disease the world has ever known. . . . By the end of 1991, just four and a half years from now, it is projected that 270,000 cases of AIDS, including 197,000 deaths, will have been reported in the United States. During 1991 alone, it is estimated that 54,000 Americans will die from AIDS." Estimates of the costs of treating AIDS by 1991 ranged from $8.5 billion to $38 and even to $112 billion.

Three Areas of HIV Concentration

The public was aware that the two leading areas of HIV concentration were New York City and San Francisco. The virulence of the epidemic in other areas of major concentration was not general knowledge—South Florida; Newark, New Jersey and San Juan, Puerto Rico—nor was there a sense of what areas of the country as yet untouched by the disease might expect to experience if AIDS was permitted to spread.

FLORIDA

Testifying before the Presidential Commission on November 12, 1987, Dr. John Witte, assistant state health officer, reported that Florida with more than 8,000 reported cases had 7 percent of the AIDS cases in the nation along with an estimated 29,000 cases of ARC and 145,000 asymptomatic individuals infected with HIV. He anticipated 32,000 cases of AIDS by 1991. Thirty-eight percent of the cases were among blacks (as against the national average of 25 percent) and 12 percent among Hispanics. Whereas the national percentage of cases of heterosexual transmission was 4 percent, in Florida it was 15—almost entirely among IV drug users, their sexual partners and offspring. Some 10 percent of the cases were among immigrants from Haiti, where heterosexual transmission played the major role in the spread of the disease.

NEWARK, NEW JERSEY

Of the 310,000 people in the city, 66 percent are black and 9 percent are Hispanic. The median age is 27. In 1988 over one-third of the population was below the poverty level, the highest percentage of any U.S. city. The unemployment rate was 20–25 percent, and 29 percent of the population received its income from government support programs. The intravenous drug abuse rate, 350 cases per 100,000, was the highest in the nation. It was estimated that 3–4 percent of the people of Newark were HIV-positive. The majority of AIDS cases (73 percent) were in the childbearing 20–39 age group. Because many of the AIDS patients were homeless or lacking family support, a disproportionate number occupied expensive hospital beds.

SAN JUAN, PUERTO RICO

A city of 425,749 people on an island of 3.2 million, San Juan in April 1988 reported 273 confirmed cases of AIDS out of 1,054 for the island as a whole. The percentage of cases among Puerto Rican women was 11.34 percent of the total as against 7 percent for the United States; and of drug addicts, 40 percent as against 17 percent. Puerto Rico was fifth in incidence of pediatric cases, with 4.3 percent of the total of

AIDS cases in the nation and with a fatality rate of 76 percent against the national rate of 58 percent. The great majority of AIDS patients, medically indigent, required extended hospital stays because other services were not available.[1]

By 1992 the Centers for Disease Control forecast 6,612 cases of full-blown AIDS for Puerto Rico, with 2,645 of these in San Juan along with 113,225 and 19,836, respectively, cases of AIDS Related Complex. The total number of HIV infected cases, including the asymptomatic, the CDC projected at 142,830 to 280,370 for San Juan (or 25–60 percent of the city's population) and 357,048 to 700,872 for Puerto Rico (or 10–20 percent of the island's population).

In the United States generally, by 1991, according to a CDC projection, 80 percent of HIV cases would be outside the 1988 centers of concentration. In addition, AIDS would increasingly become a disease of drug abusers, their sexual partners and offspring on the East Coast, Florida and Puerto Rico.

Hemophiliacs

In the AIDS epidemic, a particularly tragic, though small, community at risk is the hemophiliacs. Dr. Robert L. Janco, director of the Comprehensive Hemophilia Clinic at the Vanderbilt School of Medicine, offered the Commission the following statistics:

> 524 hemophiliacs have progressed to AIDS; 1,200 to 2,400 will develop AIDS.
> Five to 20 percent of spouses are infected. . . . Forty of the hemophiliac cases
> are under 13 years of age. . . . 11,000 of the estimated 14,000 men with
> hemophilia . . . may have been exposed [through blood transfusions] and may
> be at risk for developing opportunistic infections. . . . we can . . . project that as
> many as 500 sexual partners of hemophiliacs may develop AIDS.

AIDS and the General Social Crisis

At its first public hearings, in September 1987, Charles Rangel, a congressman representing black and Hispanic communities in Harlem and other inner-city sections of New York City and chairman of the House Subcommittee on Narcotics, exhorted the Commissioners to a broad conception of their task. He declared:

> We are in a free country that can legitimately boast about being the richest and
> most powerful and the most well endowed and blessed nation in the world, yet
> we continue to have people without jobs, people without decent educations,
> people without a place to sleep, people who have no food and no idea where
> their next meal, if they are lucky enough to get it at all, is coming from. . . . It is

---

[1] Vivian Chang, Health Administrator for Region II—New York, New Jersey, Puerto Rico, and the Virgin Islands—of the U.S. Public Health Service, states that many cases of AIDS in Puerto Rico have gone unreported because of a lack of sophistication in maintaining statistics as well as because of a lack of testing laboratories, along with an underreporting of cases due to homosexual or bisexual transmission because of Catholic condemnation of homosexuality and the tradition of machismo.

little wonder why such a sense of hopelessness and helplessness abounds in our society today, especially among our young people, who see only a dim light at the end of the tunnel we call the future. I can understand why the AIDS virus appears to be taking a heavier toll among this nation's black and Hispanic communities. AIDS and drugs are the most deadly one-two combination to hit American society in modern times, and it promises to get worse. . . . Arrogance from those of us who neither live the life style nor come in contact with the people most at risk of getting the virus would be the Roman-like Achilles heel of America. We had better realize that AIDS threatens the entire country.

In a sign of the direction in which his own response to the AIDS crisis would evolve, Admiral Watkins, at this first session still a mere Commission member, called Rangel's statement "one of the finest presentations I have heard in this field."

Admiral Watkins was not alone in becoming more and more convinced of the need for a comprehensive social approach to the AIDS crisis. At the Miami hearings on November 12, 1987, Dr. Lee commented:

When you get into these factors that underly where AIDS hits . . . into the illiteracy problem, unemployability problem, you get into the teen-age pregnancy, the single-parent households, the chronic welfare dependency—all of these types of things create people that do nasty things with themselves. They inject drugs into their veins. When you have a 25 year old person who has not gone through the sixth grade, who is a drug addict, who is unemployable, and 70 percent of these people also are carrying the HIV virus . . . you are really dealing with a terminal case. I . . . would like to see our Commission address some of these underlying concerns.

"The Admiral," remarked Vivian Chang, public health administrator for Region II,

will have to say that all these [critical social] problems are interlinked, but whether the Commission will come out with a broad statement saying that the only way you are going to cure this disease is if you take care of all of society's ills is doubtful. We've said it before about health, about education . . . the basic societal ills really are the root cause of illiteracy, low productivity, unemployment and total despair of some people, a significant group of people who for all intents and purposes don't really exist.

To fulfill Dr. Chang's injunction, the Commission would have to undergo an intensive and impelling education.

CHAPTER

First Steps in the Education of the Commission

No one of the numerous critics of the Presidential Commission could have foreseen, of course, what Colleen Conway-Welch subsequently pointed out: that as a result of their experiences on field trips and at public hearings, the Commissioners would expand their horizons, modify their attitudes and beliefs and produce a final report that would win the applause of the entire AIDS community.

The Presidential Commission began its learning experience with on-site inspections of the areas with the highest concentration of AIDS cases: New York, San Francisco and Southern Florida.

In California, the Commission encountered the most comprehensive effort against the epidemic in the nation, a model for many of the recommendations the Commission would offer in its "Final Report."

◆ ◆ ◆

Criticism of the composition of the Presidential Commission had been especially virulent in California. "Our worst fears may be realized," declared Republican Bruce Decker, chairman of the State AIDS Advisory Committee, "that they'll come up with a dreadful, Draconian, knee-jerk policy that will lead to quarantines and widespread mandatory testing. Look at the makeup of the commission, and you can imagine the worst-case scenario without too much difficulty."

The sharp criticism reflected a widespread resolve in California, unparalleled elsewhere in the nation, to spare no effort or resources in confronting the AIDS epidemic. According to the *San Francisco Chronicle* of May 11, 1987, 73 percent of

Californians believed that "AIDS is the most important issue facing the state and research for a cure should be the top priority for increased state financing."

The prompt and effective response of San Francisco and of the state of California to the medical emergency was due in great part to the aggressiveness of the gay community, particularly in San Francisco, where gay political power was exemplified in the establishment on October 27, 1985, of a twenty-four-hour vigil at the Federal Building—a continuous vigil designed to call attention to the urgency of a heightened federal response to the AIDS crisis. As the *Chronicle* noted on August 5, 1986, "In San Francisco, where homosexuals have political clout, Mayor Dianne Feinstein and the Board of Supervisors have addressed the AIDS epidemic by paying for extensive education programs, medical treatment and vigorous enforcement of a tough anti-discrimination law."

San Francisco inaugurated a $12 million municipally funded AIDS program that included an outpatient clinic and an expanded ward at San Francisco General Hospital, bereavement counseling, hospice units, houses for homeless AIDS patients, home services, social services, and city-financed chronic-care beds for people too sick to remain at home but not requiring acute-care hospitalization.

In 1985 Governor George Deukmejian signed into law an extraordinary series of bills extending the tenure of the State AIDS Advisory Committee and increasing its membership; strengthening confidentiality protections and barring the use of the antibody test as a condition for insurability or employment; and appropriating $5 million for alternative sites for AIDS testing.

In September 1985 another comprehensive bill provided $2.3 million for clinical research, including antiviral drug trials; guaranteed supervised attendant care not covered by medicare or insurance providers; funded demonstration projects to test the cost-effectiveness of in-home care over hospitalization; and provided $1 million for home health aides, attendant and hospice care and other services to patients in the acute phase of the illness and $200,000 for initiating a comprehensive study of health care costs to enable state planning for and funding of necessary AIDS treatment programs. A further $600,000 was voted for an AIDS Mental Health Program; $250,000 for education of hospital, home health agency and attendant care workers; $150,000 for an evaluation of state-funded educational programs; and $400,000 for pilot programs for education and detoxification of sero-positive intravenous drug users.

In 1985 the State Department of Health Services funded a Computerized AIDS Information Network (not to be matched by federal agencies for another four years) as well as a statewide Hemophilia AIDS Project.

In January 1987 California became the first state to promote the development of an AIDS vaccine when the state health department offered $4 million as a subsidy to local manufacturers who would undertake such a project and an additional $20 million to guarantee purchase by the state of 1 million doses of such a vaccine.

On June 26, 1987, two days after President Reagan issued his executive order establishing the Presidential Commission, the California State Assembly enacted the first comprehensive state plan to fight the AIDS epidemic, passing a bill drafted by Assemblyman Art Agnos in consultation with U.S. Surgeon General C. Everett Koop.

Convinced that neither the Reagan administration nor the Congress was about to mobilize a massive effort against a crisis that, according to estimates by state and federal officials, would bring an increase in the number of California AIDS cases from 8,938 in June 1987 to a minimum of 52,000 and possibly to as many as 187,500 cases by 1991 with a cost to the state of perhaps $5 billion, on June 18 State Attorney General John Van de Kamp proposed a state program to test experimental drugs without federal approval. On a television news program he declared that FDA had been "glacially slow with its development of drugs for AIDS. . . . You don't need FDA approval," he noted, "to actually set up testing procedures here in California."

On September 28 the California legislature passed and the governor signed into law legislation that, according to Van de Kamp, permitted "a streamlined, non-bureaucratic approach to the single problem of curing AIDS—a process overseen by a distinguished group of scientists and doctors whose task will be to cut the red tape out while leaving the scientific and medical vigor in."

In July 1988, contrasting the state action with federal lethargy, Dr. Marcus Conant, a member of the California State Department of Health AIDS Leadership Committee and the first physician in the nation to establish a hospital AIDS clinic, told a Senate committee chaired by Senator Edward Kennedy that in 1987 "within a week of passage of legislation for a State Department of Health Food and Drug Administration, Jonas Salk submitted a proposal. It was approved within a month. He had it in humans by November, and he had data to report to the [International Conference on AIDS] in Stockholm (in June 1988)."

◆ ◆ ◆

The Shanti Project

Spending per AIDS patient in Los Angeles, reported the *New York Times* on February 8, 1989, was "double that in San Francisco, which relies on volunteer agencies and non-hospital care whenever possible." Outstanding among these volunteer agencies was the Shanti project, founded by Dr. Charles Garfield in 1974. Discovering that participants in a study of cancer survivors at the Cancer Research Institute of the University of California at San Francisco, like colleagues with whom he had previously worked in the Apollo moon landing project, were "high achievers with a clear sense of mission, goal and results-oriented," Garfield concluded that "we could form a community service of substantial worth and impact" among cancer survivors, health professionals working with them and the families of the patients. He selected some twenty volunteers and trained them to become "patient advocates" or "advocate counselors." According to Garfield, "the single strongest asset the Shanti volunteer has is the willingness to walk into the emotional life of another person when invited to do so. . . . This is far less psychotherapy than it is human compassion."

When a local TV reporter asked the name of his project, Garfield on the spur of the moment replied with the Sanskrit word that means "the peace that passeth understanding"—Shanti.

In 1980 Shanti received its first AIDS referrals. A large number of those responding to a call for additional volunteers were PWAs. By 1988 a staff of fifty-three full-time and ten part-time people along with more than 600 trained volunteers organized into twenty-one support groups were providing emotional and practical home support to some 4,500 people (80 percent of the PWAs in San Francisco) with individual counseling, support groups and a practical support program along with patient counseling at San Francisco General Hospital, the city's chief AIDS clinic and research center. In addition, Shanti was providing long-term, low-cost housing for forty-eight PWAs; in 1988 Shanti opened a residence for women with AIDS and had plans for a family housing program.

Shanti became a major factor in the confrontation with AIDS in San Francisco and a model for similar projects in New York (GMHC), San Juan, Juneau, Reno, Tucson, Cincinnati and Oklahoma City as well as in Stockholm, Paris, Berlin and Brighton (England).

New York Tags Along

The summary findings and conclusions of the "Proceedings of the Public Health Service Roundtable on AIDS" in August 1987, a month before the Presidential Commission held its first meeting, declared: "The Metropolitan New York area is the global reservoir of HIV infection. Efforts to combat AIDS in this [Public Health Service] Region II area will therefore have a national and international impact." According to the United Hospital Fund "Blueprint" AIDS issue of the fall of 1987, "the city has 51 percent of [the national] AIDS cases linked solely to intravenous drug use, 42 percent of cases of women with AIDS, and 46 percent of cases of children with AIDS." In 1988 a new case of AIDS was being reported in the city every two hours.

In an investigative report published in the *New York Native* for March 25–April 7, 1985, under the headline "Horror Stories and Excuses: How New York City Is Dealing with AIDS," Randy Shilts, a San Francisco journalist (author of the 1987 best-seller exposé of national bungling and indifference in the AIDS crisis, *And the Band Played On*), quoted a "well-regarded California health official" as declaring, "If we weren't dealing with such tragedy, you'd say that New York's response to AIDS has been a joke."

In New York, in contrast to San Francisco, Dr. Mathilde Krim noted, "there are no chronic care beds, no hospices, no Meals on Wheels for AIDS patients, no clinic or ward, nothing to keep people at home instead of in a hospital. Here, you have to hospitalize people in order to do any treatment, even if it does not need to be done in a hospital. It costs ten times as much and wastes a lot of hospital resources." Furthermore, in New York, unlike San Francisco, because of the lack of centralized AIDS treatment facilities, researchers were enrolling patients in experiments only at a late stage in the disease. "By the time we get people, they are pretty much at the end of their rope," said Krim. The response of city officials to appeals for action, she said, had been "polite and interested but so far noncommittal."

In July 1983, noting that "the medical resources of governments at the federal, state and local level have not yet been effectively marshalled to fight this epidemic" and that "a program of state assisted basic and applied research in acquired immunosuppressive diseases is clearly indicated," the legislature established a State AIDS Institute with a seven-member research council and a thirteen-member advisory council composed of representatives of the public, of education and medical institutions, of local health departments and of nonprofit organizations, including organizations providing services to high-risk populations.

State appropriations grew from $5.25 million in 1983 to $16 million in 1987, a substantial portion of which was devoted to training state employees involved with high-risk groups and to the implementation of an AIDS/HIV prevention curriculum for grades K to 12. In January 1986 ten hospitals and thirteen satellite clinics throughout the state were designated as AIDS centers. In the fall of that year moneys were appropriated for a New York City AIDS Service Delivery Consortium to coordinate the efforts of twenty-four organizations in the metropolitan area that provided supportive services for persons with AIDS and ARC.

Unlike California, where AIDS was concentrated almost entirely in the gay population, in New York 50 percent of the 200,000 current or former intravenous substance abusers were estimated to be HIV-infected, 80 or more percent of whom were not receiving any treatment. The AIDS Institute Expenditure Plan for 1987–1988 targeted $1.6 million for storefront operations and street teams "providing outreach, education and referral for counseling and testing to IV drug users and their sexual partners." During a six-month period in 1986–1987, however, a mere 4,287 contacts with IV substance abusers and their partners were made by outreach staff.

As of March 1987, nearly 10 percent of adult cases of AIDS were among women. With high rates of sexually transmitted disease as well as of drug experimentation among adolescents aged 12 to 17, the danger of a rapid spread of the epidemic among the youth could not be ignored.

In April 1988 the number of new cases of AIDS among IV substance abusers in the state for the first time surpassed that among gays.

Official figures of HIV infection were clearly incomplete. According to an AIDS Institute report, "Expert opinions lead us to speculate that there are 5–10 cases of other serious HIV-related conditions that result in hospitalization for each case of AIDS recorded."

On May 15, a Gay Men's Health Crisis newsletter reported the formation of a New York AIDS Task Force including GMHC, the Association for Drug Abuse Prevention and Treatment, Family Planning Advocates, Hispanic AIDS Forum, United Hospital Fund, Federation of Protestant Welfare Agencies, PWA Coalition and the Minority Task Force on AIDS. "When the state budget was passed in April," the report noted, "it included almost every item the coalition requested."

A report of the State AIDS Institute was less optimistic. "The emergent nature of the AIDS epidemic," the report declared, "and its devastating human and social consequences demand an immediate response that is often impossible to muster through the machinery of State government."

New York City's Plan

In May 1988, in a major development in the fight against AIDS, the New York City Emergency Task Force on AIDS published a document of nearly 500 pages entitled: "New York City Strategic Plan for AIDS." Comprehensive, thorough in its detailed and practical proposals and imbued with a tone of compassion, this plan for the city with 28 percent of the nation's AIDS cases could serve as a model for cities and states throughout the nation as well as for foreign nations and, especially, for the Presidential Commission.

Drafted with the assistance of the Fund for the City of New York and under the chairmanship of Dr. Stephen C. Joseph, the commissioner of the New York City Department of Health, the document represented the collaborative effort of officials of several municipal departments and agencies and promulgated impressive policies and goals, including a goal of reaching by 1990 600,000 New Yorkers with HIV counseling and testing; increasing AIDS expenditures from $218 million to $383.5 million in a year; and providing care for all PWAs unable to secure government benefits or in need of assistance in locating housing or a long-term care facility.

The report explored particular problems in the crisis. "Some of the City's current clients," the New York City Strategic Plan for AIDS warned, "have active drug habits, have never lived alone, never managed money, or cooked or cleaned for themselves. It is not always possible to provide a home attendant because clients or friends may be using or dealing drugs in the house, putting the home attendant at risk." Even the prescription of AZT posed problems, the document noted. It "must be taken every 4 hours, even at night. Patients who are homeless or are active substance abusers often cannot follow a schedule such as this." Increasingly, too, the health services had to deal with HIV-related dementia. Patients "often exhibit unpredictable behavior and require close monitoring, putting great strain on the homecare worker in the isolated setting of the home."

Despite this impressive document—delayed a full seven years after the definition of the epidemic because public officials had been "polite and interested but . . . noncommittal"—not all was clear sailing in New York City. At the Gay Pride Day parade in June 1988 ACT UP condemned the city for providing only two clinics to care for nearly a half-million HIV-positive people, for failing to mount a municipal outreach program for minorities and for the mayor's announced intention to defund the AIDS Anti-Discrimination Unit.

In July, asserting that the gay population of the city did not exceed 100,000, the Health Department reduced its projection of AIDS among homosexual and bisexual men from 200,000 to 250,000 down to 50,000 and the estimate of New Yorkers infected with HIV from 400,000 (the estimate in the Strategic Plan for AIDS two months earlier) to 200,000.

Responding in *Newsday* on July 29, Richard Dunne, executive director of the Gay Men's Health Crisis and a member of the advisory panel of a Seroprevalence Survey being conducted on behalf of the federal government, pointed out that the department itself had previously acknowledged that AIDS cases had been significantly underreported in New York City. "Lost in the sterile debate surrounded by the unfortunate device of 'epidemiology by press conference,'" Dunne charged, "is the inescapable fact that New York City is not prepared to respond to a worsening health crisis."

Two months later, on September 1, Governor Mario Cuomo signed an HIV confidentiality law aimed at halting widespread HIV testing abuses and at encouraging testing among high-risk populations. According to the GMHC newsletter, "GMHC was instrumental in drafting the bill and in pulling together AIDS, public health and civil liberties organizations to lobby for it. It is the most comprehensive bill of its kind and can serve as a model for other states."

Nevertheless, five months later, on February 19, 1989, the *New York Times* quoted Cuomo as admitting that "the response by government and the private sector has been reactive, uncoordinated and unresponsive." The *Times* article called attention to personality clashes between the governor and the mayor and between the state and the city health commissioners as well as struggles over "turf" among nineteen agencies involved in developing the state plan. Carol Levine, executive director of the Citizens Commission on AIDS, a private agency sponsored by eighteen foundations, commented: "Moving two very large bureaucracies [city and state] is hard to do anyway, but pushing them to move in tandem is especially difficult."

Those with HIV infection were caught in the muddle.

What the Commission
Learned in New York City

The following transcripts of interviews conducted in August 1988 were, except for that with Dr. Norma Goodwin, with individuals whom the Commissioners either spoke to on their visit to New York City or listened to subsequently at Commission hearings. Engaged in the daily struggle against the epidemic, these New Yorkers gave the Commissioners a sense of the AIDS struggle as it is lived day by day.

Dr. Senih Fikrig, Professor and Vice Chairman of Pediatrics at Downstate Medical College

"Our first HIV patient," said Dr. Fikrig, who emigrated from Turkey to the United States in 1954,

> was a Haitian infant with pneumocystis, in 1981, soon after the first description of cases of pneumocystis carinii pneumonia in San Francisco. After recovering from the pneumocystis, the infant developed a massive cytomegalovirus infection and died. Someone on the hospital staff said, half in jest, "Maybe this is baby AIDS." Three years later, the father died of cryptococcal meningitis. Subsequently, when anti-body tests became available, we tested the serum of the dead father and infant as well as of the older sibling and the mother. All except the sibling tested positive. Then, at last, we were able to diagnose with certainty what the infant had had.

By 1988 Downstate and the neighboring and associated Kings County Hospital had treated 140 HIV-positive children, of whom over 100 died. Since, however, no specific test had been developed for infants under 15 months, untested infants were not included in CDC statistics even if pediatricians recognized HIV infection in them.

The clients of Downstate, which is situated at the southern end of Brooklyn, are primarily blacks and Haitians. The latter, mostly recent immigrants, are poor; they have language difficulties and are traditionally suspicious of physicians. Preoccupied constantly with problems of food and shelter, Haitians worry about health problems only secondarily.

"Some of our patients," said Dr. Fikrig, "ask whether I would mind if they also went to see voodoo doctors. I have no objection. At the moment we're not providing them with anything much better than voodoo medicine." Insofar as AZT had not been tested with pediatric AIDS patients, Dr. Fikrig had no approved medication with which to treat pediatric HIV infection. He was at the moment engaged, in fact, in a clinical test of gamma globulin.

At Downstate and Kings County hospitals, of the 7,000 deliveries annually, 2 percent (or 140) of the mothers were testing positive as well as about 50 percent of their offspring, for a total of some 70 new pediatric patients a year. Six percent of the pregnant Haitian women were testing positive.

Dr. Fikrig was collaborating "with some success" with a Haitian social worker, Marie St. Cyr-Delpe, director of the Haitian Coalition on AIDS, in seeking funding for Haitian social workers. Ms. St. Cyr was trying to promote trust in Downstate and Kings County hospitals so that the Haitians would feel comfortable about going there with their children.

What is different about pediatric AIDS? "Whenever you're dealing with the pediatric age group," replied Dr. Fikrig, "you're dealing with the whole family. If a child is positive, 99.9 percent of the time the rest of the family is also positive." Eighty percent of the children under Dr. Fikrig's care were under 5 years of age; 90 percent, under 2.

According to Fikrig, when a physician asks mothers to take care of their children, he has to realize that they have problems taking care of themselves and their husbands. The problem is complicated by the fact that many of the mothers are addicts. "I have had mothers," said Dr. Fikrig, "who behave almost violently in the clinic. They shout, 'I'm waiting here 15 minutes and no one has taken care of me.' Then they go to the lavatory and shoot up or take something, and they come out different people." In addition to their addiction, they may have other illnesses. They all have financial problems. In many instances, the mother is dead, the father is dead, or they have disappeared. Ten to 20 percent of the pediatric patients have suffered abuse from parents.

"Grandmothers take extremely good care of these children," Dr. Fikrig noted. "But, really, one should go through parenthood only once. On the whole," he declared, "our experience has also been good with foster mothers. Even the most willing foster parents, however, sometimes find they cannot handle children with HIV infection and ask to be relieved within 3 to 6 months."

Dr. Fikrig recounted how after the parents died of AIDS, the foster mother had a child, 5½ and under her care for two years, tested. The child tested positive. Although he was asymptomatic, the woman panicked. She brought the boy to the hospital and left him. A month later she returned. She couldn't live without the boy. At the moment she was in the process of adopting him. On the other hand, Dr. Fikrig pointed out, this boy was a lovable and intelligent child generally in good health. Other children were not so fortunate.

What about burnout in pediatric AIDS? "Depends on the days," responded Dr. Fikrig. "I have been in medicine for more than 30 years. I am not unfamiliar with death although I haven't treated a group before that I knew was going to die. In that sense, there is frustration, and sometimes I do experience burn out. Generally, I am reconciled to nature."

Dr. Fikrig attributed the slower response of federal agencies to pediatric AIDS to the small incidence among children as compared to adults. Children with HIV infection, he noted, do not have spokesmen for their cause because the problem is not nationwide but is concentrated in parts of the Bronx and Brooklyn in New York City and in Newark and Miami. Furthermore, these children come from addictive or poor minority families not accustomed to organizing in defense of their rights.

Recently crack had invaded the local communities. Fifteen percent of mothers on crack were testing positive. "Every day," declared Dr. Fikrig, "when we go over the admissions from the night before we find 3 or 4 crack-using women who have given birth and to more premature, lower birthweight children with small head size and inherent complications." Fikrig added ironically, "A generation of future presidents!"

Dr. Fikrig believed that the spread of the disease outside the minorities might bring a change in attitude about AIDS. "If you go to North Shore Hospital," he said, "you will see that they are treating predominantly white and middle-class women and children with HIV infection, drug addicts. They have white grandmothers taking care of children."

"The human race has survived other epidemics," Dr. Fikrig remarked. "Plague, smallpox, cholera. My hope is that it will survive this epidemic also."

Dr. Lorraine Hale and Hale House

A Vassar graduate, Dr. Hale had assumed most of the responsibilities of the children's shelter founded by her 83-year-old mother, Mary, known affectionately in Harlem as Mother Hale. In their shelter, one of a row of four-story buildings with a stoop on a quiet residential street, they have a small reception room and a dining room downstairs and bedrooms and playrooms on the remaining floors. The building was recently renovated and gives a sense of cheer and welcome.

Hale House gets referrals from hospitals, from social service agencies and from sick mothers unable to take care of their offspring. Neighbors and people in the community and even the local police direct children to the shelter. "People trust us," said Dr. Hale. "There are other choices for children in need, but people choose us because of our reputation." Indeed, Mother Hale was invited to attend President Reagan's 1988 State of the Union Address, honored as a person who was making a significant contribution to the nation.

In 1985 when Hale House received its first child with HIV infection, Lorraine Hale informed the municipal Special Services for Children (SSC) agency that Hale House was prepared to care for such babies. Not until two and a half years later, in January 1988, did she receive a reply—a negative reply. In the meantime several other child care agencies had been assigned the task.

Dr. Hale applied to the state, but state officials rejected every facility she showed them.

According to Dr. Hale, incidents where blacks are blocked by prejudice are so ordinary, so much a part of life, that people don't take notice. When she complained, for example, to SSC that she did not want a particular SSC planner (each agency is assigned one) because the girl had turned hostile and begun to sulk after Dr. Hale rejected something she suggested, an SSC official exclaimed, "What do you mean you don't want her? You have to have her." "Instead of dealing with the issue I raised," said Dr. Hale, "they wrote me a long list of complaints about Hale House and refused to let us open a home for AIDS babies. They described Hale House as 'inconsequential,' Hale House! The agency that brings them more publicity than any other in the city!"

At the moment the fourteen-member staff (rotating in shifts), most of whom were not trained professionals, was unaware that two of the infants in their care had HIV infection. It was a question whether to inform them in advance of the children's condition, as professional ethics might require, or to allow them first to become so attached to the children that they would be loath to abandon them upon learning of their infection. Dr. Hale had chosen the second option and had invited Dr. Stephen Nicholas of the Harlem Hospital Pediatrics AIDS clinic to discuss strategy. It would be Dr. Nicholas's task to reassure the staff about their safety and to outline minimal precautions.

Dr. Hale did not believe in segregating AIDS patients. "This is a home for all children," she explained. "If they come to us, we're going to keep them." If they became too ill, she would send them elsewhere. "But as long as we think we can do all the magic that you can do with babies, we're going to continue to do that. My mandate, my mother's mandate, is to see to it that these children live as full a life as they can. That means they have to be in an integrated society [that is, infected along with the noninfected], not in a place just for AIDS." She did not want people to pass on the street and say, "That's the AIDS house."

Dr. Hale was planning a home for infants with various terminal diseases, including AIDS. "AIDS to me," she said, "is a medical problem. It became social only because of the media." She was not convinced that a pediatric AIDS epidemic existed. "If in New York City we have identified only 331 children during the last six years, that is hardly an epidemic. When you identify five new cases a month, you cannot say we have an epidemic. Part of my belief is due to the fact that I don't want it to be an epidemic because it's so horrendous. I maintain a stance that will not permit it to be an epidemic."

As for the critical problems in the black community that provide the environment for the spread of AIDS, Dr. Hale declared:

> We have drug addiction, we have suicide, we have violence against each other. As white folks devalue us, we devalue ourselves, and it becomes all right to kill ourselves off. When I see a woman who is a drug addict, I see the face of racism close up. When you are constantly barraged with the idea that you are not as good, that you are not a person but a mere object, not everybody can stand up to that. And if you have to be black, for Christ's sake, at least be light and with straight hair. Or be an athlete.
>
> Who put blacks on drugs? Black folks don't grow drugs, and we don't bring them into the country. On the other hand, one thing we have never understood is that we do have choices. If all the black folks decided that they were going to give up drugs and that they were all going to college, room would have to be made for them. But as a people we have very much played into the system. I cannot simply say those folks did it to us.
>
> There needs to be a change, but there won't be a change. It's like a second Reconstruction. Racism is an integral part of the system. The victims of AIDS are the outsiders—the homosexuals, who are barely tolerated, and the blacks, who are not tolerated. You compound racism with disease, and they become the untouchables. AIDS is an excuse for further separation, but the underlying problem is greed. People are concerned with how much they can get for themselves as quickly as possible. We don't care about children. We care about things, a big car, a house. I'm not horrified that people are selling drugs. The country says do whatever you can to get rich, but get rich you must.

Dr. Stephen Nicholas of Columbia Presbyterian Babies Hospital and Harlem Hospital

Dr. Nicholas, the physician invited by Dr. Hale to prepare her staff for the presence of sero-positive infants, had chosen pediatrics as his field because he likes children, and he discovered, to his surprise, that he also liked pediatricians, whom he describes as "kids in perpetual childhood. You can't interact with kids without being gentle," he explains.

In 1981 at the age of 27, Dr. Nicholas arrived in New York from Wyoming wearing cowboy boots and "scared to death" at coming to study pediatrics at the prestigious Columbia Presbyterian Hospital. By 1987, six years later, he had achieved a sufficient reputation to be chosen to draft a significant part of the report of the Surgeon General's Workshop on Children with HIV Infection and Their Families.

When the first reports of a strange new infection appeared in the *New England Journal of Medicine*, Nicholas's reaction was "Thank God, that's something I don't have to worry about. But when it became clear that HIV was like the hepatitis B virus, often transmitted at birth, pediatricians were alerted to the possibility of pediatric HIV infection."

In 1982 during Nicholas's one-month rotation at Harlem Hospital, a child was born to an IVDU prostitute in what was the first recorded report of AIDS during pregnancy. The mother died shortly after giving birth. Although the baby looked normal, the entire hospital staff was alarmed. The infant was put in isolation, and the door was kept closed. "Everyone," recalled Dr. Nicholas,

> put on 2 gowns, 3 gowns, 5 pairs of gloves, several masks. They provided just what care they had to, feeding and changing diapers. But an interesting thing happened that shows how pediatrics is different from much that we're hearing about care for adults with AIDS. As the weeks went by, the door was kept open a little more often. People went into the room with one gown, one pair of gloves, one mask. Toys appeared in the crib. Nurses started to sing to the baby. The recognition that this was a baby who needed basic things overpowered the fears. It became everybody's kid. Each of us would hold that baby on rounds.

Dr. Nicholas commented, "If you had polled the staff during those early years, they would have said unanimously that they did not want to take care of AIDS patients. When you take opinion polls or attitude assessments, the results may bear no resemblance to actual behavior. People generally say they are lenient but behave otherwise. Here was little James Oglesby, a baby we've raised, a baby we love. We have to do what's right for him."

When Admiral Watkins, the chairman of the Presidential AIDS Commission, visited Harlem Hospital, he was taken to see little James. Watkins later recalled: "He had a wonderful smile, a wonderful face. He was a wonderful little boy, the epitome of the AIDS tragedy. These real-world cases make a difference. It's like touching a name on the Viet Nam memorial. Why do we let these things happen without getting stirred up? Why are we waiting for a social crisis to get on with these things?"

At Harlem Hospital after 1982 the number of HIV cases doubled every year. In a cost study with the first thirty-seven patients, the first such study undertaken in the United States, the staff found that it cost $3.5 million for patient care, 20 percent of which was due to the children's living in the hospital awaiting foster care. "During the early years," recounted Dr. Nicholas, "many of the children died after 2 or 3 days in the hospital, often of pneumocystis pneumonia. Infants six months of age or younger have no resistance against this opportunistic infection. Some die later, they rot, literally; the brain goes, everything goes; and they die little by little. Costs will rise when AZT is authorized for pediatric AIDS and extends life."

Dr. Nicholas shows visitors pictures of his patients. One little girl of whom he was particularly fond had arrived suffering from severe malnutrition. The mother was an intravenous drug user, 22 years old. She was selling herself for drugs and had previously had a little boy who died of AIDS. "The nicest mother, very tender." A Chinese man, 55 to 60 years of age, who claimed to be the godfather, came to the hospital every day and sat at the child's bedside and cried. When Nicholas said to him, "You're grieving more like a father than a godfather," the man confessed that he was the father. When the child died, the nurses and the staff collected money and paid for the burial. "The first of many kids we've paid for," noted Nicholas.

In 1985 at Harlem Hospital Dr. Nicholas began enrolling women into prenatal clinics. Aware that he had a very pale face for dealing with drug-using women in central Harlem, he asked himself: "How am I going to do this?" He knew they were saying, "What's this white dude doing in a black clinic?" These women were accustomed "to lousy, episodic health care—health care for poor people stinks. It's underfinanced, it's crisis oriented. There is no assumption of a one-to-one relationship with the care provider. But the suspicion broke down around the children." They came to believe him when he said: "I'm here because I care about your baby, and I'm here because I care about you." He had to be careful not to appear judgmental. "This attitude," Nicholas noted, "is hard for doctors because we're so demanding of ourselves. We want the patients to clean up their act, to get plugged into all these programs. But if you set too high a level of expectation and they like you and they fail, they can't come back to face you. My message to young physicians is what we do with our personalities is more important that what we do with our minds.

"It is the central point of pediatrics that we become the advocate for a family, for a kid and all his world. That's a revolutionary concept for IV drug using parents. We've finally got some social workers to help us, but for the longest time I was doing pre-natal counseling and all the HIV related counseling as well as all the general social services. A major contribution the government could make would be to simplify matters so that you could go to one central location and get all the various services."

A prospective study with a large cohort was under way, Dr. Nicholas reported, to identify risk factors. He believed it likely, though as yet unproven, that the children of women with HIV infection who were otherwise healthy have a better prognosis. A few infected children around the nation had reached the age of 6 to 9 and were almost entirely normal. At Harlem the doctors see only those who fall sick, and they have, therefore, a skewed idea of the effect of the virus.

Dr. Nicholas had had a running disagreement with representatives of ACT UP, who oppose the use of placebos in all clinical trials. "How," Nicholas asked, "does one design a clinical trial so that you have information that is interpretable, the best information in the shortest amount time and, hopefully, doing the least amount of harm?" The ACT UP people suggested, for example, that it was cruel to put an IV in the children in a clinical test of gamma globulin and that the infusion took inordinately long since it lasted a couple of hours. Nicholas countered that there is a significant benefit to nonmedical interventions—loving and attention. The staff assembles around the child during the infusion and provides support to the family. A nutritionist uses the opportunity to discuss problems of diet. (An infant undergoing such an IV infusion in a similar test at Dr. Fikrig's clinic at Kings County Hospital appeared quite at ease and content, happy at being the center of attention.)

"The ACT UP people," Nicholas noted, "are telling us to give the therapy without a double-blind study, but to determine whether something works we have to compare it to something. We have no historical comparison because there have not been enough infected children in one place. It's my impression that everybody looks better since we have started the test, including the parents. We're doing something."

By 1985, Dr. Nicholas declared, the hospital began to have more of another group of children like one who had recently died. The mother, "a wonderful woman," a college graduate, had a good job at AT&T. The father worked as an assistant manager in a large clothing store. They brought in a handsome little boy about 1 year of age, very thin. "I took one look at him," said Nicholas, "and knew what it was." The father had been wild as an adolescent. During 1978 he had experimented with IV drugs. He had turned himself around, however, finished high school, found work and married. He had infected his wife, and she, the baby. Invariably, Nicholas noted, we identify the baby as HIV-infected first because it has a shorter incubation period. With this diagnosis, what had appeared to be a successful middle-class existence abruptly came to an end.

"This week alone," said Nicholas, "we had one family in which a little girl of four died, the mother, an IVDU, died a day or two later, and a six-year-old sister is dying in the hospital.

"In doing research or providing care, where do you start?" Dr. Nicholas asked. "You see this disease against the horrible backdrop of poverty and isolation and IV drug abuse with HIV added into the equation. In middle-class communities generally there are family support groups, there is someone the sick person can talk to, to share with. I think the statement, 'I'm an IV drug user' says it all."

The first time Dr. Nicholas visited Hale House was to reassure the staff about Kenyatta, a beautiful little girl about 3 years old. Despite his advice, Kenyatta, who had no symptoms of infection, was transferred to a hospital. Kenyatta's mother, an IVDU, had died of tuberculosis. The father, a tall, strong, good-looking man, had won admission into Phoenix House, a drug rehabilitation center, to break himself of alcoholism and a drug habit. Eager to show her brother support, an aunt took Kenyatta in. Immediately, boyfriends, friends and family ceased coming to visit her. She was also taking care of her grandson's twins, a little younger than Kenyatta, and was always worried about their becoming infected. After Kenyatta's father had been out of Phoenix House for about a month, he resumed his drinking. His sister refused to bear the burden of his child any longer. Another sister, irresponsible and unpleasant, took Kenyatta. One day Nicholas received a call: Kenyatta had been drowned in the bathtub. The sister's lover had resented the child. The crime was never investigated.

Dr. Nicholas disagreed with Dr. Hale's denial of the existence of a pediatric AIDS epidemic. "It's an epidemic," he insisted.

> In parts of northern Manhattan and the South Bronx, 4 to 5 percent of all
> newborns have been exposed to the virus. You can say that in certain areas it's
> endemic, not epidemic. In Baltimore, New Haven, Newark and Washington,
> there's an epidemic. You can pretend that it's not an epidemic when it is

concentrated in a particular segment of the population, as it is, among the inner city poor. It hasn't reached Paoli, Pennsylvania, Westchester or Long Island. But it is the most common diagnosis we make. In Harlem Hospital 120 babies will be born this year HIV positive out of 3,000—4 to 5 percent. In certain areas, a whole group of children are going to die. Since mothers are not routinely blood tested, we don't know how to interpret the data based on the number of ill kids that we've got. There's preliminary evidence to suggest that as a woman progresses from asymptomatic to a disease state she's got more virus and is more likely to transfer it. The rate of infection continues to double annually and has shown no signs of slowing down.

When people speak of a third wave of the disease [first gays, then IVDUs], they mean male to female and female to male transmission. What they really mean is, when is it going to show up in Westchester? We don't know whether it has. The incubation could be going on now if it has spread from the underclass. Incubation may take longer in individuals with fewer co-factors. A healthy Westchester individual who has a fling may not get sick for 8 or 10 or 15 years—unlike the original group of promiscuous homosexuals that had previously had all the 22 sexually transmitted diseases.

In August 1988 Dr. Nicholas had just lost a bottle of sherry in a wager with his superior, Dr. Margaret Hagearty, because they had finally succeeded in overcoming bureaucratic red tape to establish a shelter for AIDS babies.

The biggest single problem at the Harlem Hospital Pediatrics AIDS clinic was the children living at the hospital because they had no other place to live. Initially, Drs. Hagearty and Nicholas had discussed the possibility of Lorraine Hale's establishing such a home as an adjunct to Hale House, but after a year had passed without movement Dr. Hagearty learned of the availability of an abandoned convent.

Phase I of the plan was to get the children out of the hospital environment. Phase II was to recruit foster parents from among volunteers who would help at the convent and might want to take children home. The convent could accommodate twenty-five children, who would be organized into four families, each with its own name—the tangerine family, the apple family, and so forth—and with two care workers serving as parents for six children along with nurses and social workers and Dr. Nicholas as medical director.

To win the goodwill of the community, the two physicians enlisted the aid of the pastor of the local church, a member of the community board in the predominantly Dominican community. A doctor on the hospital staff, a Dominican who lived in the community, helped make other contacts. They introduced themselves to the local fire chief and had a long visit at the 34th Police Precinct. They asked for police visibility at certain hours because crack is widely sold in the neighborhood.

The police captain called his community advisors to sit in on the discussion. "What you're doing is very important," they said. "We can't spare much manpower, but we'll do what we can." Since the Harlem Hospital staff conducts an outreach program for schools, the police suggested names of parent-teacher activists who could be helpful. Of the community they said, "These are poor people. Crime is the biggest worry. Your biggest problem is going to be the 'crazies.' Just let people know what you are doing."

Dr. Iris Davis at Woodhull Hospital

Iris Davis, the AIDS assessment coordinator at Woodhull Hospital in the Bushwick section of Brooklyn, is proud of the fact that she is the daughter of a black migrant worker who put himself through college and worked his way up to becoming an Army officer. Her father and her mother, a schoolteacher, were always involved in community activities.

While conducting a project in West Virginia during her medical education at the University of Virginia at Charlottesville, Dr. Davis became aware that race was not necessarily an issue in health care, but economics certainly was, and culture had a great deal to do with medical services. Desiring to train as a primary care internist in the inner city, she went to Montefiore Hospital Center in the Bronx and then to Harlem Hospital. She completed her education on a Public Health Services grant.

As early as 1981 the staff at Harlem Hospital was reporting to the Centers for Disease Control signs of the HIV infection. Gay Related Immune Deficiency Syndrome (GRID), as the disease was then called, was supposed to end at 34th Street in midtown Manhattan—that is, confined within the gay community. "We could tell them that we were seeing cases of heterosexual transmission."

When Dr. Davis was assigned to work in a general clinic and became a community-based practitioner, she saw HIV infection in an ever-larger spectrum. The patients were not addicts as society views addicts, that is, as someone totally dissociated from regular life. "There is a tremendous level of a drug problem not perceived or dealt with," said Dr. Davis, "among people who work and function productively." In her opinion, the figure of 40 million Americans taking drugs regularly or sporadically is an underestimation inasmuch as the term drug abuser generally does not include the numbers of people who shoot up on New Year's Eve or at other parties and drink so much as not to remember with whom they then went to bed. "People with whom I work," Dr. Davis said, "wonder, too, how much an underestimation there is in the figures of HIV infection inasmuch as there has not been adequate anonymous screening to arrive at a proper estimate."

At Woodhull Hospital in the Bushwick section of north Brooklyn, the staff had been searching for months for a coordinator for the hospital's AIDS program, and in mid-July 1987 Dr. Davis was offered the position. In setting up a culturally sensitive HIV program, Dr. Davis dealt with all the hospital departments, successfully with some and not so successfully with others. HIV infection among women with genital infections, for example, was a major problem, but the obstetrics-gynecology department was more than 50 percent understaffed.

According to Dr. Davis, HIV infection must be treated with one-on-one therapy. "We have only five people on our staff," she pointed out, "but we've been able to have an impact much beyond the 537 people on our present patient load. [Additional patients were referred to other hospitals] because we interact with the families and the families interact with the community. 'You've got HIV,' we say to a patient. 'We don't know how much time you have. We'll keep you on the best therapies we can get. In the meantime you start to change the community so that the problem will not recur with your children.' If you don't have that attitude of building on weakness," comments Iris Davis, "then you can just sit down and die."

Woodhull has a cross section of New York City within its patient population: 20 to 25 percent whites, predominantly gay or bisexual; more than 30 percent Hispanics; 25 percent American blacks and the remainder Haitians or Caribbean blacks. Many of the patients are or were formerly substance abusers.

Woodhull attracts a number of middle-class black patients because they feel more comfortable with a staff that understands how hard they had to struggle to get where they are only to have it all destroyed by HIV. One current patient delayed marriage for fifteen years because she and her husband wanted to work themselves out of poverty first. After marriage they discovered that the husband had infected the wife. They were both sero-positive. She suffered from recurrent tuberculosis. He was becoming increasingly stressed, trying to support a sick wife and two children.

"We're seeing great-grandmothers called upon to provide support," says Dr. Davis. "How is the State going to confront further devastation of support structures in low income communities? We deal with a lot of these issues at the New York State AIDS Institute, but there is no response."

A large percentage of gay men of color claim to be bisexual and have relations both with men and with women. "It is important," says Dr. Davis, "when you start discussing sexual partners to be specific. If a patient informs his single long-time partner, the wife, will he inform the four males with whom he has flings?"

The Woodhull staff conducts an outreach program, each member taking turns in accepting speaking engagements. "We tell people they cannot assume if they are black or Hispanic and sexually active in New York City that they have had no contact with HIV. That's a hard message until you say, 'I want every twentieth person in the room to stand up,' and then say, 'That's how many are already infected.' Next you say, 'I want one in 7 to stand up.' Only then do they start asking questions."

In the general patient population, Dr. Davis advises women to be tested. She tells them that they cannot know where their husbands have been. The testing has revealed high statistics—one in every three or four women positive through sexual transmission, asymptomatic. Although Dr. Davis recognizes that her sample is small, "the percentage among New York women," she says, "is certainly not one in 20, as CDC claims, and even that percentage is frightening, especially among women in childbearing years. What is the actual rate in a community like this one? No one knows." The Woodhull staff hoped to obtain money from CDC to do a sero-positive study in the hospital emergency room.

On February 15, 1989 the *New York Times* reported that a testing of blood samples of 143 emergency room patients at the Bronx-Lebanon Medical Center in

July 1988, with known AIDS patients excluded, showed that 23 percent were infected with HIV. Similar high rates of infection were found in another study in the South Bronx at Lincoln Hospital.

In addition to all the other problems, Dr. Davis points to institutional racism, a health care system in which a low-income person is not comfortable, to which he or she has no access and no coping strategies. "Suppose a woman calls the clinic and says, 'I haven't anybody to take care of the babies. I've got mine, my sister's and my next door neighbor's, and nobody's getting back until 2 o'clock, and I have to get more AZT today because I'm running out.' What you must say is, 'Is it too many kids to put on a bus?' If the woman says no, then you say, 'Bring all the kids and leave them in the day care center down the hall.' If you lack that understanding and tell her to get a babysitter or simply say that this person doesn't fit in the structure, then you can't provide health care to such a woman."

The hope lies, according to Dr. Davis, in the rebuilding of community structures destroyed during the Reagan era. Although organization is taking place in black and Hispanic communities in New York City, it is not happening fast enough. Blacks look at AIDS as just another plague. In the past there were tuberculosis, syphilis, poverty. "This may be the last plague for many of us," she declares. "Only drugs have brought similar devastation. This is the greatest crisis facing people of color now. If we don't learn how to talk to kids who are attracted to street life, if we don't teach women not to have kids early in life and not taking responsibility for them. . . . If our society is not set up to examine some of the societal ills that predispose people to behaviors that make them susceptible to HIV, then where do we start?"

Nationally, Dr. Davis says that since the Reagan era public health services, especially in the urban areas, had been devastated. Ten years into the epidemic, she charges, there have been no sero-positive studies, and no current test can expose a virus that hides in macrophages (a portion of the cellular nerve system).

The New York City public hospitals system has been pushed past its limits. "You see administrators walking out of hospitals, saying 'I just don't think we can take any more cuts and honestly pretend we're providing health care.'" Homelessness and poor home environments are complicating factors.

> You can't expect families to accept an AIDS patient in a home where there are three babies down with salmonella.
>
> This disease could wipe out every major city in the nation, and I wouldn't be surprised if that happened on the basis of the current national effort to control it. We still don't have public health counselors in New York City, where the fastest rising rates are in heterosexual transmission. There's no money for people to track down routes of transmission in the communities and to explain the necessity for being tested and being tested early.
>
> For some portions of our society, it is too late. How do we say to a man dying of AIDS, "Don't go home to your great-aunt in the South and have a relationship with the woman next door?" You can't change behavior unless you are willing to change other aspects of lives. How do you help a Hispanic gay

man to accept the fact that he is gay, to understand that he has a spectrum of sexuality within his life?

We are working against an epidemic that does not give us time. We no longer can say that racism will be gone in another generation, we no longer have time to say that we will settle the issues of medicare, homelessness and equity.

Dr. Norma J. Goodwin, Bedford-Stuyvesant Youth AIDS Prevention Project

Dr. Goodwin hardly looks her 51 years. "I'm active and the activity keeps me young," she says. In 1961 Dr. Goodwin came to New York to complete her residency and internship. At Downstate Medical Center she became clinical director and then director of the artificial kidney center, serving with Dr. William Kolff, inventor of the artificial kidney. Over the years she became frustrated at the lack of humanity with which patients were treated and the lack of privacy and dignity and efficiency in the care, and her interest switched to public health service. "I think there is something wrong when a person has to go to x-ray and is forced to wait first in the emergency room for four or five hours, is tied up at x-ray for a couple of hours and then waits 7 or 8 hours to find out whether a bone is broken. What goes on in many hospitals wouldn't be tolerated at a General Motors or an IBM plant. In the health field we need to be good managers but not become heartless and lose a sense of humanity about what we're trying to do.

"We have a class system in the country," Dr. Goodwin insists. "The poorer you are, the less good the services you are going to receive."

Unlike Dr. Hale and Dr. Davis, Dr. Goodwin did not immediately mention racism in relation to the quality of health service. "I would be derelict," she declared, however, "if I did not do so. There is a correlation in this country between economic status and race, and blacks and Hispanics bear a disproportionate brunt of the lack of caring in American society. That the AIDS epidemic is disproportionately attacking those populations is a reflection of their problems generally."

Dr. Goodwin herself had had intense experiences with racism. In the mid-1950s, when she was applying for admission to medical schools, her mother and father were indignant that she did not include colleges in Virginia. When she responded that a black would never be accepted in a southern white college, her mother, a schoolteacher, exclaimed: "You were born in Virginia, we are Virginia residents, and you have as much right to apply to those schools as anybody else."

During a grueling admissions interview at the Medical College of Virginia in Richmond ("very intimidating for an 18 year old," Dr. Goodwin recalls), the dean asked her in a broad southern drawl, "What do you think about the race problem?" "I looked at him and said, 'It's very simple. I believe the right will triumph.'"

After acceptance at the Medical College, Dr. Goodwin's problems were not over. Although she was not the first black to matriculate there, she was the only black student and one of four women at the time. She was totally isolated, without friends, often the victim of cruel humiliations.

"Had I gone to a black college," Dr. Goodwin says, "I would not have had such negative experiences at a young age. It is possible that I became a stronger person as a result."

In 1977 Dr. Goodwin gave up most of her duties at the Downstate Medical College to establish a public health service agency—AMRON (Norma spelled backwards) Management Consultants, "a management consulting firm which provides a comprehensive range of services, programs and systems aimed at maximizing the effectiveness and efficiency of organizations, including institutions, businesses and governmental agencies." Among AMRON's numerous and prestigious clients are agencies of the Department of Health and Human Services, state health agencies, colleges and universities, and hospitals.

In 1984 Dr. Goodwin obtained a grant from the National Cancer Institute to develop a health information and promotion service to decrease the incidence of cancer morbidity and mortality in the black community. AMRON formed Health Watch, whose sole mission was cancer education and prevention. "The black population," she discovered, "experiences so many negatives, especially the economically disadvantaged segment, who wants to hear about cancer?" Dr. Goodwin expanded the scope of the Health Watch activity to include hypertension, heart disease, diabetes and obesity. "We call these the major black killers, responsible for almost 80 percent of excess black deaths."

In 1985 Dr. Goodwin had an experience close to home when a young man who had worked at AMRON before moving to a job at the City Health Department died of AIDS. From then on she began hearing of more and more cases.

In June 1987 the advisory council of Health Watch decided to make AIDS the agency's top priority. A month later, at the CDC Conference on AIDS and Minorities in Atlanta, a representative of the National Conference of Mayors mentioned to her that the mayors' conference was offering a grant. Applications were due four days later. Dr. Goodwin rushed back to New York and worked nonstop, almost without sleep, to complete the application. She obtained a grant of $20,000.

On October 25, 1987, Dr. Goodwin organized a conference at Downstate Medical College under the title "AIDS in the Black Population—Clinical, Health and Political Implications." Many national experts were in attendance. All but two of the speakers were black. "We don't usually think of having many black experts on AIDS," Dr. Goodwin noted.

Instead of an anticipated audience of 150, 400 people attended, including some 100 physicians—all black—other black health professionals, nurses, social workers and technicians as well as 50 medical students from Downstate Medical College and several dozen community people.

With the grant from the National Conference of Mayors a program was developed targeting teenagers, and the Bedford-Stuyvesant Youth AIDS Prevention Project (YAPP) was organized, one of the most structured youth AIDS prevention efforts in the country. An immediate objective of YAPP, according to the prospectus, was to develop brochures providing "accurate, relevant, culturally sensitive information on AIDS"—one directed to teenagers, "The Real Deal about AIDS"; and another, "Your Teenagers Don't Have to Get AIDS," for parents or guardians of teenagers.

The project planned to establish focus groups for pretesting educational materials.

> It is a major problem that we assume that we know what the young people know, think and want. In the teenage brochure, for example, we said that AIDS was more common in the black than in the white community. We thought it was important for the young people to know that they were at increased risk. The young people objected. They felt somehow it was a discriminatory statement.
>
> Our long-range objective is to get peer counselors from among the teenagers as well as from among the parents. There's such a stigma attached to AIDS that Health Watch has not yet sought to involve PWAs.

At the Conference on AIDS organized by Health Watch, however, Dr. Goodwin had a photograph taken of her embracing a person with AIDS. "It is important," she says, "to keep showing people that AIDS can't be spread by casual contact."

Health Watch aimed at the establishment of a community advisory group composed of youth, parents, and representatives from the schools, the health sector, the religious sector and the community at large. "It's hopeless to talk to teenagers in a vacuum," Dr. Goodwin advises. "We have to look at their environment, and there are teenagers and teenagers. You can't use the same approaches with 11 and 12 year olds that you use with those 17 to 19. At first because we didn't have enough resources to work with all the teenagers, we decided to work with those less likely to have become sexually active to prevent infection among them." With funding from the New York State AIDS Institute, however, Health Watch was subsequently able to expand its activities to include teenagers from 15 to 19.

After money was obtained from the Centers for Disease Control to replicate YAPP in Harlem, Newark, Philadelphia and Baltimore, Health Watch began working with local agencies in those cities.

AMRON conducted a symposium on black adolescent pregnancy under the sponsorship of the Empire State Medical Association. Of this problem Dr. Goodwin declares that

> adult America, not the adolescent is a major part of the problem. When the additional external influences adolescents are exposed to—which range from parents and significant others' exhibiting sexually explicit behavior with multiple partners, to the highly suggestive recurrent messages carried by the media . . . —there should be no surprise that the incidence of unplanned adolescent pregnancy is approaching epidemic proportions. . . . that economically disadvantaged, unemployed, often undereducated adolescents who are by definition, culturally and socially deprived, are more vulnerable to conflicting adult messages and external pressures for immediate gratification.

As for the related problem of drug abuse, Dr. Goodwin declares:

We can't afford to use a different set of values with IV drug users than we use
with a rich movie star who is able to buy and use cocaine or professional people
who abuse tranquilizers. The problem relates to crime because the majority are
poor. These people are using their resources to get their drugs just like a doctor
or professional without a problem in getting drugs. We have our own Third
World within the United States.

As to the general perspectives in the national AIDS crisis, Dr. Goodwin declares:

What the AIDS epidemic has done is to highlight fundamental problems which
have existed in our society, which, for whatever reason, we've put on the bottom
shelf and refused to confront. In order for society to grapple successfully with
the myriad of problems caused by the epidemic, we must address many
fundamental problems which we have tended not to want to address. The
tragedy is that we have let them get so far out of hand—the drug abuse problem
and out-of-wedlock pregnancy. As a physician, I refuse to accept that nothing
can be done. . . . The IV drug user is at the bottom of the ladder. Rather than
looking at why that person is there, society doesn't give a damn. With the
continuing vestiges of racism, clearly there are many who won't give a damn as
long as the epidemic is just in the black and Hispanic communities. It is myopic
to assume that a contagious disorder can be contained within a particular
population. . . .
    When you consider the kind of effort that would be involved in making
structural changes, you can understand, given the deterioration that has taken
place, why it's unlikely there's going to be the willingness to make those
changes.

Dr. Wilma Bulkin and the
Beth Abraham Hospice

An oncologist (specialist in tumors) at Montefiore Medical Center in the Bronx since
1967, Dr. Wilma Bulkin, who is 51, grew up during World War II "with all its death."
Her generation, she says—today's leaders in the medical profession—sought to deny
death, and with the development of antibiotics and medical technology they could
do so. Before the war, doctors could cure few diseases. Comfort and consoling were
part of their training and responsibility. In Dr. Bulkin's generation, people went to
medical schools to learn to cure, and the other aspect of medicine was neglected.
    Dr. Bulkin had an early experience with death when at the age of nine she lost
her father. In the early 1970s, when her mother was dying of cancer, she shared the
nursing with her sister, traveling from New York to Philadelphia on weekends. "A
lot of people in hospice work," she says, "have experienced death, and it helps." As
a cancer specialist, she came to the realization that most of her patients were dying
and to accept death as natural, but she still needed to learn how to care for the
terminally ill.

The first conference of the National Hospice Organization took place in Washington in 1978, attended by 2,000 people from all over the United States and Canada—legislators, hospice theoreticians, social workers, clergy, hospital administrators, and physicians. Following that meeting the president of Montefiore, who had first espoused the principle of home care in the United States, set up a task force to define whether a hospice was needed in the Bronx. The task force decided that a hospice did not belong in a hospital inasmuch as a hospice is a program not for curing or for investigative medicine but only for care. Thus it was placed in Beth Abraham, a nursing home adjunct to Montefiore. Dr. Bulkin was appointed director.

Medicare regulations adopted in 1983 set parameters for hospices: patients' life expectancy of six months or less with no benefit from further curative therapy; receipt of 80 percent of care at home with a caregiver assuming responsibility for the custodial care and for decisions in the event the patients ceased to be competent.

Initially, hospice care was set up almost solely for cancer patients, for whom, unlike cardiac and other patients with life-threatening diseases, a prognosis of death can generally be made with some accuracy.

At a conference in 1984 Dr. Bulkin was impressed by the contention of Elisabeth Kübler-Ross, author of the influential book *On Death and Dying*, that a hospice that did not accept AIDS patients had no right to be called a hospice. A year later, in consultation with the administrator and directors of the hospice, Dr. Bulkin reached the decision to include AIDS patients in the hospice program. Immediately, requests for admission arrived from all over the city, but a limit of 10 percent of the total patient population was set for AIDS patients.

A hospice, Dr. Bulkin explains, is a multidisciplinary program for provision of care of the total patient during the last six months of life. It is a *program* of care, not a particular place. At Beth Abraham twenty-five staff members along with volunteers run the program—nurses, social workers, administrators, homecare managers, patient coordinators, admissions coordinators and in-patient coordinators. A lot of coordination and management is required for the unit of care, which in hospices, unlike in acute-care settings, is not simply the patient but the patient and family. The general quota for the Beth Abraham hospice is thirty-five patients, but because of the constant turnover, the hospice accommodates about 275 patients a year. During 1986 and 1987, about sixty AIDS patients were cared for.

To become knowledgeable about HIV infection, Dr. Bulkin joined the Montefiore AIDS team. She learned much, she says, from the patients themselves. As an oncologist, she had seen Kaposi's sarcoma in 75-year-old Jews. (It is a disease common in elderly Jewish men, rarely in the young.) Since this disease is not found among IVDUs with HIV infection, the typical AIDS patients at Montefiore, Dr. Bulkin spent time investigating the latter at St. Vincent's Hospital in Greenwich Village, where most of the patients are gay.

AIDS cases, says Dr. Bulkin, pose special problems. The patients are generally younger. (The Beth Abraham hospice has dealt with AIDS patients from 23 to 65, and even one of 72.) With some of the IVD abusers, the families are also drug abusers and cannot provide home care for patients. Often children are involved. Drug abusers with AIDS typically have a manipulative adolescent personality. The staff become their parents, setting standards and imposing discipline, often with strict controls. Dr. Bulkin has seen drug abusers grow up quickly in their last months. "Death is nature's way of making us grow up," she notes, quoting Woody Allen.

In the February 11, 1988 issue of the *New England Journal of Medicine*, Dr. Bulkin in collaboration with Herbert Kukashok of the Albert Einstein College of Medicine published an article entitled "Rx for Dying: The Case for Hospice." In the article the authors sum up the problems in hospices, "the most appropriate and humane [environment] . . . for caring for the dying patient with AIDS":

> The stress and frustration of being unable to cure patients with AIDS may lead physicians to refer them to hospices prematurely; the life expectancy of AIDS patients may often be underestimated so that the six-month life-expectancy requirement cannot be precisely determined; caring for patients with AIDS may exacerbate the stress on care givers because they are dealing with dying patients their own age; shifting the identification of hospices to AIDS could affect the way hospice care is viewed by other patients and by their families and physicians.

In her testimony before the Presidential Commission, Dr. Bulkin estimated savings of over $500,000 at Montefiore through in-patient hospice care instead of in-patient acute hospital care.

Dr. Bulkin rejects the general practice of hospices throughout the country of catering almost exclusively to middle-class patients and their families. The social problems of the poor, she believes, are so overwhelming that they have greater need of the program. At Beth Abraham the multi-ethnic composition of the staff is a factor in the success of the program. She herself, she says, has always been emotionally involved with her patients. "I care about them. I make sure they're getting the kind of quality care they should have."

As hospice medical director, Dr. Bulkin made the rounds of the patients. At weekly team meetings, at which each patient was discussed from an interdisciplinary point of view, it was her responsibility to offer a prognosis of each patient's condition and to discuss current and future medical and physical problems. The team drafted a plan for the death and helped with funeral arrangements. A psychiatrist met with the team regularly on the common problem of burnout. New hospices, according to Dr. Bulkin, experience considerable staff turnover until routines are established.

Dr. Bulkin herself has experienced burnout from her zealous advocacy of hospice. "It is considered anti-establishment," she says. "I wanted it to become establishment right away. I wanted people to understand that death is a reality and that to give false hope to people is wrong." In the hospice the patient is encouraged to express fears of death in discussions with the doctor and the staff. Almost everyone, according to Dr. Bulkin, comes to a point of reality. "We try to make it a peaceful, comfortable death."

Physicians have often transferred the care of terminal patients to the hospice and ceased all connection with them. "Wilma, you take over," they say. In the *New England Journal of Medicine* article, Dr. Bulkin comments: "Physicians will continue to be uncomfortable in the hospice context until their training prepares them for the realities that not all disease can be conquered by intervention and that pursuing every means to prolong life, regardless of its quality, is doing no service. Even as we teach them to cure, we must teach them how to care for those they cannot cure."

"AIDS," says Dr. Bulkin, "is exposing the current problems in medicine, particularly in the training of physicians. If a physician does not know how to deal with death and dying and doesn't want to learn how to do so, how will the problem be handled? The time of denial of death is coming to an end. We have to learn how to take care of the dying."

In January 1988 Dr. Bulkin resigned as medical director of the Beth Abraham Hospice. "Career women," she explained, "have to make a choice between career and family. With my husband retiring, I could not continue with the kind of emotionally involving work that I was doing. I still go to the Montefiore AIDS team meetings as often as I can. I go to the hospice once or twice a week. A young man that I trained has taken my place. He hasn't experienced death in his family, but he's good."[1]

Gordon Hough, Administrator, Bailey House

In 1975, unable to find a position after obtaining a doctorate in English literature, Gordon Hough studied heroin addiction treatment. For a year and a half he administered a drug abuse clinic in Buffalo and then for nine years one in New York City. Subsequently, he worked in a program for "street kids" in Greenwich Village. With this background he was well qualified for appointment in June 1987 as administrator of Bailey House, a shelter for homeless people with AIDS that had been established six months earlier.

Following a September 1986 Coalition for Lesbian and Gay Rights and Lavender Hill Mob camp-in at the mayor's Gracie Mansion residence (organized by Mobster Mike Petrelis, subsequently a resident of Bailey House) and a demonstration outside Bailey House, the city opened the residence before a full staff had been hired. The building was filled one floor at a time until the maximum of forty-four residents was reached in July 1987. In August 1988 twenty-two of the residents were black, a dozen Hispanic and another twelve white, with the percentage of minorities constantly growing.

"Our goal," says Hough, "is to help people live with AIDS rather than die from it. Some residents don't want to do anything but lie down and wait for death. Others survey the scene cautiously for a week to a couple months and then become involved

---

[1] The hospice was subsequently discontinued for lack of funds.

in the residence council, in growing plants, in volunteer activities, in helping other residents sicker than they or in visiting people in hospitals."

Arts and crafts are offered on Monday and trips on Thursday. Tickets are distributed for all kinds of events. Residents are given stipends of up to $65 a month for working in the building. Some engage in volunteer work elsewhere.

Referrals to Bailey House come through the City Division of AIDS Services, which periodically sends over a stack of intake applications. The Bailey House staff, which can accept no more than five or six new people a month in place of those who have died, evaluates the applications and selects a number to put on a waiting list. Clients come from hospitals, where some have been hospitalized for years, and from hotels and YMCA residences; PWAs who have lived in single rooms and now require more support or even just a private toilet.

The Bailey House staff of some forty people is divided into a maintenance corps and a support team, which includes a social worker, a social security counselor, a part-time social worker who does intake, a social worker assistant, a recreation therapist, an educator who deals with specific AIDS issues and with hygiene, a nurse practitioner handling medical treatment and personal care assistants. For clients no longer able to carry on daily living chores, a visiting nurse serves as a home health care worker.

"Many PWAs served by organizations of the gay community like GMHC," says Hough, "are hardworking, tax-paying, well-employed, conventional individuals. That's a feature of AIDS that makes the epidemic seem so poignant." On the other hand,

> Many of the persons with AIDS at Bailey House cannot be characterized in those terms. Indeed, for the people at Bailey House AIDS exists in a wider context of need. They are homeless with little familial support, with limited incomes and resources and very likely with histories of poor health. They have either had many different jobs or a limited employment history although a few with good employment histories lost everything through prolonged hospitalization.
>
> Often families do not want to cope with persons with AIDS. One day a woman brought her sister from Long Island to Bailey House and left her at the front door, exclaiming, 'Now don't come back.' The woman had had a laryndectomy and been fitted with a voice box, which she used ineffectively. She had left school after the 7th grade and was desperately in need of services and care. Bailey House rejected her as a possible resident because the staff could not deal with a person with whom they could not communicate. She was sent back to her sister and died shortly afterwards.

Three recent young residents—19, 22 and 24 years of age—had been living on the streets as prostitutes with no family and no friends. At first they had a stream of visitors, acquaintances from the streets, but when they became weak, nobody came to visit them. "The staff," according to Hough, "is not large enough to deal with such people, who need a more structured, more psychiatrically oriented setting."

The staff has had to adjust to the fact that persons with AIDS do not "sprout wings and catch a halo. We found out what people's needs were," says Hough, "and devised structures. We discovered, for example, that people were uneasy when guests simply popped in. Many who had lived in SROs [single-room occupancy hotels] experienced drug dealing and violence and were uncomfortable at outsiders wandering about. Now guests have to be cleared before they are admitted into the building."

Dementia, a common disease among AIDS patients, poses special difficulties. Residents with the disease walk about aimlessly; they light cigarettes, set them on the bed, and light up another. Health care workers must watch them around the clock, even sitting up all night outside the door.

Staff burnout is a problem. "AIDS is an illness," declares Hough, "which causes people to deteriorate gradually. It's very hard for people committed to helping others to see that despite the help they're giving, people are becoming weaker, thinner and sicker. Everyone's special person does die. Death," says Hough, "is difficult for the staff to deal with, and twice a week the staff assemble in support groups to discuss issues of stress."

With an average of a death a week at the house, individuals are always dying. Some residents have left because they could not cope with the bereavement.

Satisfaction for the staff comes in seeing residents who are happy or at least less unhappy than they had ever been before. One fellow who was failing fast received a visit from his mother, who had never traveled outside her rural Georgia county. When she got out of the bus in New York, it was like "landing on a moon of Jupiter." The recreation therapist organized a trip to Coney Island. The man and his mother went on the merry-go-round. It was the greatest thing that had ever happened to him. He died a week later.

Another resident, Steve, who scarcely spoke during his first month at Bailey House and was resentful when people insisted upon greeting him, was moved to a hospital in serious condition. His case worker discovered that his mother, whom he asked to see, had died three weeks earlier in a nursing home. An inquiry revealed that the mother's body had lain in a morgue for three weeks awaiting identification. The Bailey House staff arranged for her burial. Steve died shortly thereafter, and the staff buried him at her side, as he had requested. Then Steve's father appeared. He had been living in shelters, homeless and bedraggled. Hough arranged to get him into a residence where he could be washed, clothed and fed.

Hough estimated that 2,000–3,000 people with HIV infection were living in mass shelters, many of them undiagnosed. (Other estimates ranged as high as 4,000.) Those who come down with opportunistic infections are hospitalized and housed in SROs upon discharge. Often, unhappy with their quarters, they run off and disappear. Hough doubts that these people are included in Centers for Disease Control statistics. "People are not yet dying on the streets," Hough declares, "but they will be.

"What have I dealt with this week?" Hough exclaims. "I can't even remember." At the end of last week we dealt with a resident who was going out of his mind. This week a member of the staff learned that one of his children was infected with HIV.

Then there was a suspicion that someone was dealing drugs to his room." (Such an offense is punishable by expulsion.)

Hough was not optimistic that funds would continue to be available as HIV infection increasingly became an underclass epidemic. "Our society," he declares, "tends to reward ambition, greed, success and narcissim, to use a psychiatric term, rather than service and commitment to those in need. Everybody's going to church every Sunday is not going to bring the reestablishment of family ties that never really existed."

As for drug abuse, Hough says that solutions were not to be found in Nancy Reagan's "Just say no!" buttons, but in providing treatment upon demand and jobs. A solution, he suggests, emphasizing the depth of the current crisis, might be found in universal conscription after high school with the Armed Forces teaching everyone to read and write.

"It is my opinion," says Hough, "that when capable people study the problems, regardless of their political persuasions they are going to come up with remarkably similar solutions. I don't think, however, that anything like a comprehensive solution is likely."

Hough's observation about arriving at similar solutions despite ideological differences, as will be seen, proved accurate in regard to members of the Presidential Commission.

Jack Kells of Covenant House

Jack Kells is public relations director for Covenant House, a shelter for runaway youth in New York City's Times Square area founded by Father Bruce Ritter. One night, thirty years ago, Father Ritter, a member of the Franciscan Conventual Minor Order engaged in pastoral work on the Lower East Side, heard a knock on his door. Two young people who had just been filmed for a pornographic movie had no place to stay. Father Ritter took them in for the night. After searching in vain during the next two weeks for an agency to take care of the runaways, he decided to establish a shelter on his own. Eventually he moved the shelter to Times Square and established six other smaller shelters in Manhattan. Altogether they were accommodating about 12,000 young people every year.

A television reporter in Houston, Jack Kells did a story about Father Ritter and then invited him to Houston to assist him in opening a center there. In Fort Lauderdale, a district judge weary of sending runaways to jail learned of Father Ritter's work and organized a center in her city. Other centers were founded under similar circumstances in New Orleans, Houston, Anchorage, Toronto, Antigua, Guatemala, Honduras and Panama.

Funding from New York City, New York State and Federal agencies together provided about 5 percent of the total income for the Covenant House New York operations. The general budget came from 600,000 contributors donating $2 to $10 a month.

The centers conduct an extensive national public service campaign on television, broadcasting an 800 telephone number for runaways to call for referral to the nearest shelter or agency. Word of mouth among runaways brings others to the shelters. In addition, members of the staff go out into the streets to meet young people.

Kells declared:

> We get all kinds of kids, wealthy kids and the very poor, all living on the street. We get them as young as a day old and up to 21 years of age. [In August 1988 Covenant House had seventy pregnant young women in residence.] Some stay an hour, some a day, some a year. If a kid is fairly undamaged, and there's a family to send him home to, we can get him out of Covenant House in a matter of minutes. Those who have been on the street for only a few days generally can be returned home. With those who have been runaways for more than a month a return home is less likely, and those who have been on the streets for at least six months will probably never go home. If they've been on the streets a year or more, the probability of their surviving yet another year is slim.

If runaways have no place to go and they're underage, they can stay at Covenant House for a long time—even years. At Covenant House, the runaways learn about living and about themselves and go into a long-term care program called "rites of passage," which includes mastery of job skills. There is a public school within Covenant House. Many go on to college. "We're proud," says Kells, "of those who have gone from living on the street to working on Wall Street."

On the streets runaways survive on prostitution, selling drugs, hustling, odd jobs and mugging. They live in subways, in abandoned buildings, on rooftops, in all-night movie houses or in the parks. In New York City 70 to 80 percent are black or Hispanic; in Houston, 20 percent; in Florida, 10 percent; and in Alaska, 70 percent are Native Americans.

Most of the New York runaways are from the city. Generally, their families have disintegrated, or they don't know where their parents are. Families split up after losing their apartment in a fire or after the father loses his job. The mother may have a drug habit and no longer be able to care for her children. "We often get kids," says Kells, "who create their own family unit. The eldest brother or sister may enter a life of drug dealing or prostitution in order to send the others to school. These kids are trying to cling to some sense of normality while the world around them is burning."

According to Kells, AIDS among the 30 to 40 percent of runaways involved in full-time prostitution is devastating. (The percentage of those selling themselves simply for a night for a place to sleep is much higher.) The young runaways become infected sexually rather than through needles, with an equal percentage among young women and young men.

Tony, a Hispanic, was an example of a runaway who had contracted AIDS as a male prostitute. He became homeless when his mother went to jail. He did not know his father. At 13 with no other way to keep alive, Tony hustled at the docks. He came to Covenant House when he was 17. Within weeks his life was returning to normal. He was going to school, keeping appointments and progressing remarkably. Suddenly he developed symptoms of HIV infection and died. With the certainty of immortality that characterizes youth, the other residents refused to believe such a fate could be theirs; but Tony's death was also a shock to the staff, who had great hopes for him.

Covenant House was setting aside two floors for forty young PWAs. Kells was convinced that the nation did not appreciate the AIDS crisis among young people. "If the disease is an exotic in most of the country," Kells warns,

> it won't be long. Our kids travel. Kids from New York end up in Ft. Lauderdale, they hitchhike all around the country, and as they travel they're sleeping with people. If CDC speaks of 700 teenagers with AIDS, they must all be here in New York City.
>
> Everybody is studying them, talking about them, but I've got them. I've got to house them somewhere. Two years ago in AIDS research teenagers were an anomaly. Two years ago we started to get them, now we've got more. By the time they get around to figuring it all out, I'm going to wonder whether I'll have any floor space left. We're getting them 16 or 17 years of age. Because they're constantly reinfecting themselves, they have a short incubation period.

During the summer and fall of 1988 Covenant House began tabulating the testing of runaways of both sexes who passed through the shelter. As of October 28, 1988, of 1,111 runaways tested, seventy-four or 6.67 percent tested positive, that is, 7.42 percent of the males and 5.41 percent of the females. Among 298 Hispanics, 9.06 percent tested positive; among 190 whites, 7.89; and among 598 blacks, 5.3. Among males the percentages were 10.85 (212 tested) for Hispanics, 10.16 for the 128 whites and 4.61 for the 347 blacks. Percentages rose with age from 2.78 percent among those below 16 to 10.45 among 20-year-olds (16.88 percent among the 77 Hispanics), 7.69 percent of the females and 11.58 of the males. The figures show a far higher ratio of females to males with HIV infection than in the general population and an increasing percentage with age, except for the anomalous 11.76 percent among whites 16 years of age. It is apparent that the extent of the infection among runaways is critically disproportionate to that among the general population.

What hope did Kells have that the nation would be able to resolve the AIDS crisis?

"I don't know," Kells replied. "Like a soldier in World War I, I am so deep in the trenches, I'm so busy baling out the trench, I can't see the big picture. All I can see is that the numbers are not going down. It's beginning to overwhelm us, taxing our ability to stay viable financially. It's scaring me. I worry about feeding the kids tomorrow, and the day after tomorrow is at the outer rim of my thought."

According to the *New York Times* of October 2, 1988, "a study by the Coalition for the Homeless estimated there were 20,000 children under 18 living on [New York] streets." The national estimate is over 1 million runaways at any given day throughout the United States.

Two years after the interview with Jack Kells, Covenant House was rocked with a scandal that threatened its survival. Father Ritter, accused of various serious charges, was forced to resign.[2]

Operating as a Roman Catholic institution, Covenant House fails to promote educational programs for safe sex and the use of condoms. Preaching abstinence to young prostitutes obviously provides no answer to the spread of the epidemic that alarms Jack Kells.

---

[2] In 1990, accused of various crimes, Father Ritter resigned as head of Covenant House, and the organization underwent a radical reorganization.

The Commission's Preliminary Report

$\mathbf{T}$he publication on December 2, 1987 of the Commission's "Preliminary Report," straightforward and businesslike, effected a decisive change in the Commission's public image and evoked at least tentative praise in the AIDS community. In tone and style the report reflected the influence of its military chairman, as is apparent in the following excerpts:

> The central concerns of the Commissioners will be: to eradicate the silent spread of the virus; to provide consistent, appropriate and compassionate care for those who need it; to develop strategies to locate necessary resources; and to do everything necessary to encourage research.

> It is the firm belief of the Commission that there is much to be done, that too much time has elapsed and too many people have become afflicted while questions remain unanswered.

> The need to set aside prejudice and fear in favor of compassion and a renewed sense of personal responsibility will be the challenge to leadership. . . . We must commit ourselves to the open and effective education of our citizens, as has been undertaken by our private sector volunteers, educators and public health workers.

The report announced the appointment of a Physician Review Group to be composed of clinical and research physicians of recognized HIV expertise "to advise the Commission . . . on problem-solving when addressing specific medical and research issues"; and a Health Sciences Review Group to be composed of "clinicians and scientists . . . each of whom has made major contributions within the fields of HIV treatment or research."

In an introduction to the report Admiral James D. Watkins noted that during the prior three months the Commissioners had heard testimony and received presentations from more than 200 individuals, "most of whom were AIDS patients . . . volunteers and staff of community-based and religious organizations, providers, and local, State and Federal Government officials."

At hearings the Commissioners obtained an intensive education in the problems involved in confronting the AIDS epidemic. They heard a stream of such impelling statements as the following:

> The greatest failing in the Federal response to the AIDS epidemic is our inability to mount a widespread and effective information and public education campaign, which, in the absence of a vaccine or treatment, is the only available prevention strategy. . . . There is a lack of coordination among the agencies working on AIDS education as well as overlapping programs and competing interests in the research activities being carried out by, and funded by, the various Federal agencies.
>
> —REPRESENTATIVE TED WEISS, CHAIRMAN, SUBCOMMITTEE ON
> HUMAN RESOURCES AND INTERGOVERNMENTAL RELATIONS

> [Authorities] estimate that the illicit narcotics business in our country is over $130 billion. We have 600–700 thousand heroin addicts in our country, not to mention the millions of cocaine abusers and those who abuse amphetamines and other narcotic substances.
>
> —REPRESENTATIVE BENJAMIN GILMAN, MINORITY LEADER,
> SUBCOMMITTEE ON NARCOTICS

> A generation of physicians were trained in an atmosphere of complacency. With the discovery of penicillin and other vaccines, the assumption was that the major infectious diseases could be cured or eliminated through vaccination programs. With the HIV epidemic, physicians were shocked back to the historical mainstream—they can diagnose, counsel and comfort patients and their families but seldom can cure. . . . The epidemic has challenged the profession to deal with previously tolerated inadequacies particularly in education and delivery systems.
>
> —DR. ARTHUR FOURNIER, AHEC PROGRAM DIRECTOR,
> UNIVERSITY OF MIAMI

> The cost of caring for AIDS patients (perhaps $18 billion in 1991) could topple the private insurance industry . . . and the public sector is not prepared to handle this.
>
> —DR. DANIEL SECKINGER, CHAIRMAN, FLORIDA MEDICAL
> ASSOCIATION TASK FORCE ON AIDS

> Printed materials are ineffective when dealing with groups having high illiteracy rates.
>
> —DR. SPENCER LIEB, AIDS PROGRAM SUPERVISOR, FLORIDA STATE
> AIDS EDUCATION OFFICE

The decisive message witnesses conveyed to the Commission concerned the absence of national leadership in the struggle against the epidemic. At the November 24, 1987 hearings of the Commission, after listening to spokesmen for the American Medical Association and the Institute of Medicine of the National Academy of Sciences, Admiral Watkins defined as the three most frequent issues posed in over 200 presentations: why European countries were ahead of the United States in combating the epidemic; why California found it necessary to establish a state FDA; and why PWAs receiving drugs through clinical tests complained that their friends were unable to get on the same protocol.

At February 1988 hearings Herb Spiers of ACT UP—one of a series of AIDS activists who would impress the Commission with the clarity, force and pertinence of their remarks—decried "a leadership vacuum in the fight against AIDS. Despite the noble intentions of political and bureaucratic functionaries," he warned, "AIDS will remain a controversial issue on the national agenda until the chief executive of our country removes it from partisan and ideological politics by personal moral example and by bold leadership. We have been told that AIDS is the nation's number one health problem, yet this four letter word was not once uttered in President Reagan's State of the Union address in January."

At the same session, Gerald Massinghoff, president of the Pharmaceutical Manufacturers Association, concurred that there was "a need for a forum where government, academia and industry can meet to assess the progress in the battle against AIDS, to resolve problems as they emerge and thoroughly discuss all relevant issues." The nominee of his association "as uniquely qualified" for such a role was not one of the agencies of the Department of Health and Human Services but rather the Institute of Medicine (IOM) of the National Academy of Sciences.

Massinghoff's praise of the IOM was not unjustified. In 1986, a year before the appointment of the Commission, the IOM "identified as a major concern a lack of cohesiveness and strategic planning throughout the national endeavor." In the summer and fall of 1987, recognizing that Federal Public Health Service agencies were not about to take the initiative, IOM conducted national conferences on the development of AIDS therapies and of an AIDS vaccine. So successful were these conferences that IOM established a Roundtable on the Development of Drugs and Vaccines against AIDS "to spur programs in the discovery, regulation, legislation and clinical application of measures to stem the epidemic." Representing the AIDS community among the fifteen members from "government, the pharmaceutical industry, academia, clinical medicine, the legal community and the public" were Martin Delaney, co-director of Project Inform, and Barry Gingell, medical consultant for the Gay Men's Health Crisis.

◆ ◆ ◆

Gay activists testifying before the Commission were surprised at the sympathetic reception they received. Staffer Frank Hagan, who was in great part responsible for the invitations to gay witnesses, singled out the experience of Jim Sammone, the

Orlando activist. In his prepared statement, Jim took the offensive against what he considered to be "a bunch of Republican appointees who were not going to accomplish anything." Before Jim was called to testify, however, Tom introduced him to Colleen Conway-Welch, Dr. Burton Lee III and several other commissioners. Jim said to Tom, "They're all so nice. My testimony is a little harsh." Subsequently, in reading his statement, whenever he came upon an inflammatory sentence, he lowered his head, dropped his voice and rushed through the passage. In questioning him, Lee and Welch made such comments as, "This is a good idea . . . this is what we need . . . we were wondering what was going on here." Jim was accorded a half-hour in the discussion period, more time than any other witness.

Father Fred Tondalo, a gay activist from Fort Lauderdale, had a similar reaction to the Commission.

> We treated them as fellow human beings, people that were learning. We taught them. They understood and received what we were saying. They asked good questions. We were impressed with their humanity. We were especially impressed by Admiral Watkins because of his openness. He asked probing questions and listened attentively to our responses. Dr. Primm was interested in the IV drug question and was impressed with the way we were dealing with the special problems of the minorities. Crenshaw did not seem homophobic at all. During the visit of Commission members to Fort Lauderdale, she hugged the AIDS patients and then didn't run to the bathroom to wash her hands.

In a preface to his testimony at a February hearing, Martin Delaney, never one to flatter government officials, generously admitted his previous error of judgment about the Commission: "Some of you may be aware that I was one of this Commission's harshest critics when it was first formed. I had some strong comments to make in the media, and I must say that since that time I have had to eat my words, and I have been quite impressed by the fairness and objectivity with which you have proceeded."

Bill Bahlman and the ACT UP Contribution to the Commission's Education

After the founding of ACT UP on March 10, 1987 the Lavender Hill Mob increasingly coordinated its efforts with those of the new organization and, finally, early in 1988 dissolved as a separate group. In September 1987, upon the appointment of the Presidential Commission, former Mobster Bill Bahlman found a new area of involvement. Bill's first contact with a member of the Commission occurred during a seventy-two-hour, day and night ACT UP demonstration at the Sloan Kettering Memorial Center in New York City. Without noting that his appointment to the Commission was going to be announced on the next day, Dr. Lee sent his assistant Peggy Dufour to invite representatives of the demonstrators to discuss their demand for quick approval of various alternative therapies. Bill, Marty Robinson and Jane

Elizabeth Glass accepted the invitation and had a discussion with him at lunch. "It seemed to me," recounted Bill, "that he was reaching out for help and seeking contact with us. We arranged other meetings."

At the first hearings of the Commission at the end of September, Bill, who was among the witnesses giving testimony, was dismayed at the incompetence and lack of direction and knowledge among the Commissioners. He suggested that the Issues Committee of ACT UP set up a subcommittee to monitor the Commission, with each subcommittee member assigned to investigating, meeting and following the positions of a member of the Commission. It soon became apparent, however, that the burden would have to be assumed by a single individual, and for the next nine months Bill devoted himself to this task.

According to Bill, ACT UP pressure was instrumental in persuading the Commission's initial chairman, Dr. Mayberry, to resign. At a meeting he addressed in New York City, Mayberry was roundly booed by AIDS activists. He became convinced that by continuing at his post, he might jeopardize the reputation he had won over many years. Indeed, the Commission decided to hold hearings in Florida in advance of those originally scheduled for New York out of fear of activist pressure in the city.

As Bill Bahlman's testimony at the Florida hearings demonstrated, the Commissioners' fears were not unjustified. Speaking as a member of the Lavender Hill Mob and of ACT UP, Bill announced:

> I come here today with anger. . . . You [Commissioners] should know that your lack of abilities as individuals and collectively as a Commission is just a symptom of how inadequately the federal government . . . has been responding to AIDS. . . . I have met with most of [the officials in the White House and in the agencies of the Department of Health and Human Services involved in the crisis and in the Congress]. I've heard them speak, and for the most part they make me sick. We see their lack of direction and leadership as a means of genocide.

Bill attended all the subsequent hearings of the Commission, traveling from city to city, coast to coast. Before each hearing, he studied the topic to be investigated, made suggestions to members of the staff and discussed issues with individual Commissioners. In addition, he briefed activists in each city on pressure tactics and helped to organize chapters of ACT UP where they did not exist.

"My first goal," Bill declared, "was to stop Commissioners from doing harm, and my second was to move them to do good." He learned whom to approach in particular among the staff and the Commissioners. Staff members and Commissioners accepted him as a permanent representative of the AIDS activists, and his absence was noted if he arrived late at hearings (especially because he wore a "Silence Means Consent" T-shirt). The staff made available to him, at his request, unedited copies of testimony. Bill regularly reported to the Issues Committee of ACT UP and relayed the committee's suggestions and reactions to the Commission's staff.

According to Bill, executive director Polly Gault was the brains behind the Commission. She appointed a staff composed primarily of women, top-notch organizers. They were primarily responsible for the Commission's achievements. Bill himself became a kind of unofficial staff person as well as someone who kept the Commission under scrutiny. He submitted questions to be asked of witnesses.

Before the February 1988 hearings in New York City on Treatments and Clinical Testing Bill had a two-and-a-half-hour meeting with Watkins during which he presented the ACT UP agenda in regard to FDA and NIH. Watkins, Bill reported, agreed in principle to all the points Bill made.

Bill argued at length with Frank Lilly and finally persuaded him as to the necessity of investigating research issues. At a meeting where a heated discussion took place about issues raised in ACT UP flyers, members of the Commission glanced at Bill to see his reaction. Because of his pressure and encouragement the Commission dealt with many issues they might otherwise have ignored.

By the spring of 1988 the Commission had heard from 450 witnesses. According to Tom Brandt, "no matter what Commission members were thinking or believing when they joined, they were getting educated and were going to be changed."

Interviewed on March 23, 1988 Dr. Lee insisted at first that because of his private practice experience with AIDS patients, nothing had surprised him in the Commission's hearings and site visits. After a half-hour of discussion, however, Lee admitted: "A lot of material has been thrown at us. I knew a lot going in, but I know ten times more coming out."

Interviewed on April 15, Colleen Conway-Welch said: "If this horrible experience does anything for us, I expect that it's going to identify solutions to the problems that those with AIDS, the chronically ill and those needing long-term care generally are going to face. I think that AIDS is the catalyst forcing a lot of examination we would not have attempted otherwise."

The proceedings of the Presidential Commission on the Human Immunodeficiency Virus Epidemic did, indeed, usher in a new stage in the struggle against the epidemic. Not only did the Commission provide a new tribune for the expression of grievances and proposals from the AIDS community, but it investigated a vast range of social, economic and political problems that the AIDS community had barely explored. National discussion of the epidemic took on a new seriousness with reportage on the Commission's hearings and with interviews with its chairman.

With its December preliminary report the Commission had in hand a planning document that set the goals and procedures of the Commission and established the order of the topics to be investigated. The report provided, according to Brandt, "a superb organizational focus."

CHAPTER 14

The Crisis in Health Care Services

In the Final Report, toward which the Commission's investigations were directed, the Commissioners would not be able to equivocate about the national crisis in health care. All witnesses echoed or expanded upon the testimony of Esther Chachkes, director of social work services at the Columbia Presbyterian Medical Center in New York, who expatiated on how the epidemic had "high-lighted all the difficulties and problems of our health care delivery system. Current social, health and medical programs are fragmented, with gaps and discontinuities in services. The patient has to conform to the system rather than the system shaped to fit the needs of the patient. In particular, persons with AIDS, because they are generally young, dying and burdened with stigma, require a system that individualizes their care and protects them." She noted the broader significance of the health care crisis in the compromising of "the quality of life for all citizens when we are unable to provide adequate care for a vulnerable segment of our society. Sick people who do not receive the health care they need strain the resources of our entire social welfare system, and our neglect of their care diminishes the well being of our entire society." In an eloquent appeal, she challenged the Commission to exploit the opportunity afforded by "our experience with AIDS . . . to reexamine our attitudes and priorities and to develop models of service that legitimize coordinated comprehensive continuity of care, an approach that all illness demands. In this regard," she declared, "AIDS has become the paradigm for socially intelligent, caring response."

Hospitals and Medicaid

Testifying also at the January 13, 1988 Commission hearings, Dennis Andrulis, vice president for research and policy of the National Association of Public Hospitals, set his focus of the effect of the epidemic on the public hospital system of the nation. "Sixty-four or one percent of public hospitals nationwide," he told the Commission, "treated an estimated 17 percent of all AIDS patients during 1985," at an average loss of $6,400 per patient per year, a loss greater than for other medical-surgical patients. With an average of 25 percent of these AIDS patients having no insurance and 62 percent covered by Medicaid, "hospitals in states with restrictive Medicaid eligibility lost over $7,400 per patient per year. . . . The safety-net hospitals are also most likely to suffer the harshest consequences of this situation as evidenced by inadequate financing, inability to attract and maintain high-quality medical staff and the sheer inundation of AIDS/ARC patients. Continuation of the status quo . . . will cripple these institutions, especially as this epidemic escalates."

In areas where AIDS had not yet reached epidemic proportion, the Commission learned of problems of a different order. Joel R. Gray, a student of nursing at the University of Iowa with AIDS Related Complex, reported that fifty out of eighty Iowa institutions responding to a recent survey expressed unwillingness to accept patients with AIDS on the basis of an Iowa statute that forbade health care facilities to "knowingly retain a resident who is in an acute stage of alcoholism, drug addiction, mental illness, or an active stage of communicable disease." "In Iowa," according to Gray, "[clinical] drug trials are inaccessible or, for the most part, non-existent, and for people who are unable or choose not to take AZT there are no alternative therapies or treatment."[1]

---

[1] In September 1987 Congress voted a one-time, nonrenewable $30 million grant to fund AZT purchases. On August 24, 1988, the New York Times reported that a failure to renew the federal grant would "jeopardize the ability of 6,000 patients around the country to continue receiving the treatment, which may prolong their lives." According to the Times, health officials in California, Texas and Florida were already barring new applications for AZT. (The Congress did renew the subsidy for another year.)

In April 1988 Jeffrey A. Beal, one of eight physicians in Tulsa, Oklahoma, "who are providing collectively . . . probably 90 percent of all care rendered to AIDS in [the] community" (he himself was treating eighty to eighty-five asymptomatic patients and fifteen in more advanced stages of the disease), complained to the Weiss Congressional Subcommittee that for persons unable to tolerate AZT the nearest alternate treatment evaluation unit was 500 miles away. According to Beal, "patients cannot travel such a distance as frequently as the clinical tests require, they can't afford the expense, they can't take off from work without losing their jobs, and with their jobs, their insurance coverage without which they are not acceptable in an ATEU." As a result of these factors, the average life expectancy of an AIDS patient in Oklahoma, Beal declared, "is five months. When doctors ask patients why they have delayed in seeking treatment before developing full-blown AIDS, they look at us and say, 'What could you have done?' In the past it seemed that our answer was AZT, [but with the high failure rate of AZT,] now our answer is, 'possibly nothing.'" The growth in the number of cases of HIV infection in Oklahoma (245 as of March 19, 1988), Beal declared, was due in part to individuals "who have come home to die." Beal himself was averaging three calls a week from such people. Indeed, these "returnees" from the major centers of infection posed a threat of a spread of the disease throughout the nation.

The absence of any safeguard of confidentiality provided a major problem in Oklahoma. Patients

Crisis in Medical Personnel

In San Francisco, Dr. Michael J. Clement, coordinator of in-patient AIDS services at the University of California at San Francisco, informed the Commission that a major problem in the crisis arose from a shortage of physicians willing "to care for large numbers of terminally ill young patients, inadequate reimbursement for time spent caring for these complex patients and probably from a degree of fear for infection with the HIV virus."

Dr. Gerald Friedland of Montefiore Medical Center confirmed Dr. Clement's observation in regard to New York. "The care of the majority of the [New York] patients who are in the private sector," said Friedland, "are in the hands of fewer than 20 physicians [who] have taken on the burden of caring for the vast majority of individuals in the private sector. . . . This pattern in New York and San Francisco," he warned, "is likely to be replicated in every United States city and community in the future."[2]

Nurses

Testifying before the Presidential Commission, Helen Miramontes, chairperson of the American Nurses Association AIDS Task Force, cited a projection made before the AIDS crisis by the Department of Health and Human Services of "a 40 percent undersupply of professional nurses by 1990." An article in the American Nurses Association, Inc. "News" entered into the record of the Commission noted a critical shortage in the Middle Atlantic and Pacific regions of the nation—areas where the AIDS crisis is most acute—and pointed out that "the vacancy rate for registered nurses in United States hospitals more than doubled between 1985 and 1986, up from 6.3 percent to 13.6 percent [and] 83 percent of hospitals reported vacancies in 1986, compared with 65 percent in 1985. Of particular concern," the statement continued, "is the fact that a great percentage occurs in specialized units such as intensive or critical care, which require advanced education and skills"—units of critical importance in the treatment of AIDS patients.

Vivien De Back, project director for the National Commission Nursing Implementation Project, blamed the nursing crisis in part on Reagan administration cutbacks in health services. Her Commission, she told the Presidential Commission,

---

did not present themselves at the early stage of the disease because they feared public exposure. "There is no retribution," Beal declared, "against physicians, hospitals, institutions, employers within the state of Oklahoma for testing individuals without their consent and reporting their names to the health department. . . . At the same time," Beal added, "we are not educating the public about the symptoms and signs on a global basis or on a local basis to urge them to come in."

2 Although the American Medical Association adopted a resolution forbidding refusal of treatment to patients infected with HIV, in the 1988 Update of "Confronting AIDS," the Institute of Medicine cited a survey of 258 physicians in New York City that revealed that 25 percent "believed it would be ethical to refuse treatment to an AIDS patient." The IOM report commented: "Should such refusals . . . become more routine, the effect . . . on the health care delivery system could be profound."

was recommending a reinstatement of lost federal funds for nursing education to increase the supply of baccalaureate and higher degree nurses to act as case managers for AIDS patients.

Dentists

"For people with AIDS dental care can be an urgent need," asserted Dr. Edward Barrett of the University of Detroit School of Dentistry in testifying before the Presidential Commission, "because . . . a seemingly minor infection can trigger a life-threatening systemic illness." He pointed out that not only did some dentists refuse treatment of AIDS patients "out of ignorance and/or fear," but that "at least one dental malpractice insurer has excluded from coverage any claim arising from HIV-related dental treatment."

Fight Back in Dallas

The Commission's hearings proceeded in an environment of increasing media attention to aspects of the AIDS crisis. The PBS television show "Frontline" of June 7, 1988, for example, devoted a major segment of a program entitled "Who Pays for AIDS?" to the insurance problem in Texas, a state ranking forty-eighth in Medicaid payments. In Texas, the program noted, a person with a Social Security disability check of more than $360 a month is ineligible for Medicaid, and there is no provision for "spend down" to that limit through the purchase of drugs. As a result, most of the patients at Parkland County Hospital in Dallas are charity cases.

"Frontline" quoted Parkland's chief administrator as saying: "Here comes AIDS on top of a reimbursement system that's really sick. . . . Medicaid . . . used to cover 67 percent of the poverty population [now] covering 37 percent. . . . why would we presume that we would take better care of patients with AIDS than . . . pregnant women and children? . . . this is . . . the straw that broke the camel's back." In some cases $800-a-day hospital stays, he noted, could be replaced by $140-a-day hospice care or by home care, home nursing, home attendant care and homemaker assistance, but no money was available for such alternatives. The result, according to the Dallas hospital official, is going to be "gut-wrenching decisions here, while other people are sitting around talking about the problem."

The AIDS Clinic, where 700 of the city's 1,150 AIDS patients were being treated, was staffed by one full-time doctor three days a week, an additional doctor one-half day a week, two full-time physician assistants three days a week, four full-time registered nurses three days a week, and one full-time social worker five days a week. On July 28, 1987 the hospital restricted allocation of AZT to a maximum of sixty eligible persons at a time; other patients for whom AZT was prescribed were put on a three-month waiting list.

Questioned by "Frontline" about the health care service problem, Dallas County Commissioner Jim Jackson expressed little concern for those with HIV infection, declaring: "I can sit here and tell you that based on the method of transmission of AIDS my chances of getting AIDS are nil. . . . my chances of getting cancer or heart disease are much, much greater. And there are a lot of folks around that'll tell you the same thing. . . . it's a matter of priorities."

Omitted in the "Frontline" coverage was an account of the struggle mounted by the Dallas gay community against the very conditions described in the report.

In June 1985 the Dallas Gay Alliance (DGA) in association with the Foundation for Human Understanding, a human rights organization, established the AIDS Resource Center for AIDS education and as a referral service. Subsequently, the two groups organized a food bank along with an AIDS Financial Assistance Fund. On the morning of December 21, 1987, during a demonstration outside the city hall protesting the failure of the city government to provide funding against the AIDS epidemic, DGA drew 600 chalk figures, representing the number of deaths from AIDS in the city.

That action provided the impetus to further militant action. Early in January DGA met for three hours with Parkland Hospital officials seeking an explanation for the cancellation of the appointment of eight additional doctors to the hospital's AIDS clinic. Later that month in response to the apparent reluctance on the part of Parkland to administer PCP prophylaxis to its 500 AIDS patients, the AIDS Resource Center began to provide AIDS patients with aerosol pentamidine. On January 25 members of the Gay Urban Truth Squad picketed a meeting of the Dallas County Commissioners Court, charging that the county was failing to provide enough money for the treatment of AIDS patients at Parkland.

Three months later, following upon a three-and-a-half-hour meeting with leaders of DGA, officials of the University of Texas Southwestern Medical School announced that since no federal money under the ATEU program had been assigned to Dallas, it would embark on its own program of AIDS clinical research. In addition, the school promised to assign an additional eight part-time physicians to Parkland's AIDS clinic within thirty days. DGA leaders commented that the new emphasis on research sounded "very promising," but William Waybourn, the organization's president, added: "We wish it had happened two or three years ago."

On May 6 the hospital administration admitted that it had failed to meet the target date for increasing the number of doctors in its AIDS clinic. Hospital officials also announced that seven AIDS patients had died while waiting to receive AZT. The DGA accused the hospital of "criminal negligence."

On May 19 DGA brought suit in state district court against Parkland Memorial Hospital. Listed as co-plaintiffs were the seven patients who had died while awaiting treatment with AZT. On May 20 Judge John Marshall ruled in favor of DGA, granting a temporary restraining order mandating the hospital to end its practice of putting patients who were eligible for AZT on a waiting list. The judge also ordered a hearing within thirty days to determine if a special master, requested by DGA, should be appointed to oversee Parkland's AIDS-related services.

Early in June the hospital ended the waiting list on AZT and agreed to make aerosolized pentamidine available to three patients by June 20. (During June DGA's AIDS Resource Center provided pentamidine treatments to seventy-two PWAs.)

On June 17 the *Dallas Morning News* reported that Dr. Daniel Barbaro, who retired in May as director of Parkland's AIDS clinic, had declared in a hundred-page sworn deposition in support of the DGA complaint that Parkland could have acquired AZT at no cost from the Texas Department of Health but had failed to do so because Parkland officials felt they lacked staff to administer that drug or aerosolized pentamidine. Barbaro charged that the hospital's waiting list for AZT was "immoral and unethical." He pointed out that whereas San Francisco General Hospital had twenty-two full-time physicians, sixteen nurse practitioners and a support staff to handle 1,800 patient visits a month, at Parkland he had been the only full-time doctor attending 700 AIDS patients.

An amended complaint alleging violation of the equal protection clause of the Fourteenth Amendment was filed on July 1 by DGA in conjunction with the American Civil Liberties Union (ACLU), the National Gay Rights Advocates and other organizations. In the suit they sought "to include as a class any or all HIV positive persons, estimated to be 28,000 people in Dallas County, who 'have been and are being denied access to medical treatment at Parkland Memorial Hospital.'"

Bill Rubenstein, an ACLU attorney, was quoted by the *Dallas Morning News* on July 2, 1988, as declaring: "What we see in Dallas is a microcosm of what we fear may be happening throughout the 1990s in the country, which is the shirking of responsibility on behalf of the public hospitals and people who have the duty to care for indigent sick people." Ben Schatz, attorney for the National Gay Rights Advocates in San Francisco, called the federal case "unique" among attempts to secure medical treatment for AIDS patients. "Many people across the country," he said, "will be looking to the case as an inspiration to challenging the treatments they are getting. It could signal a new trend."

On January 2, 1989 Irvin Riddle, 33, died, the second to die among the five individual plaintiffs who filed the original suit in May 1988. "Irvin was our best witness," said Judith Levin of ACLU. "He was so affable. You knew the court was going to like him and feel for him. We could very well go to trial and not have any surviving AIDS patient to testify."

The *Morning News* quoted another plaintiff, Bill Seals, as saying that he had to face up to the possibility that the lawsuit would outlive him. "I try not to think about that, but it's a reality. If this [case] follows the normal course of things, it could take years. I don't think I'll ever see the case settled."

In February 1989 the hospital moved for a dismissal of the complaint on the basis that all problems posed by the plaintiffs had been corrected. Although the plaintiffs would have preferred to have the judge continue to supervise the hospital's AIDS services, he did dismiss the case. "Nevertheless," asserted ACLU's Rubenstein, "the case, which received wide publicity in the national hospital community, did put all hospitals on notice that they could not treat AIDS patients differently from other patients. It was a victory against discrimination with national implications."

CHAPTER 15

FDA and NIH at Bay

At one of the Presidential Commission's initial hearings in September, Cardinal O'Connor, whose diocesan institutions were engaged in the care of hundreds of New York City AIDS patients, pressed Gary Noble, Public Health Service AIDS coordinator, for answers regarding "the exorbitant cost" of the single approved AIDS drug, AZT. The Cardinal remarked on the monopoly control of the drug by a corporation that refused to produce records on the actual cost of production or on the use of federal funds in its development. "I think," he concluded, "there is either going to have to be some approach to bringing about a sharp reduction in the cost or the government is going to have to fund this to another significant extent."

Dr. Theresa Crenshaw pursued the question with Noble, asking what options there were for an ultimate reduction in the cost of AZT and for preventing a similar situation from developing with other new drugs. Admiral James Watkins followed with the observation that inasmuch as the government and taxpayers had paid a sizable contribution to the initial stages of drug development, a flat or amortization regime in the form of a lower cost of the drug seemed appropriate, especially in the special context of the current crisis. Noble responded: "I would say that given the free enterprise system as it exists now, the options are either that there is funding by government, by the private sector, by insurance; or the drug isn't available."

Commenting generally on this problem some weeks later, Commissioner Dr. Beny Primm noted: "There are people in this country who need to be represented in the drug power consortium so that when decisions are made, it is not after the fact, to have to accept those decisions ex post facto but to be part of the making of those decisions. I think that that is why I [the sole black on the Commission] am here and that is what we need in this country—the representation of all people, if possible."

These observations were incorporated into the Commission's preliminary report published early in December. On December 16, 1987, at a hearing in Federal District Court on the complaint brought the previous June by the National Gay Rights Advocates et al. against the Department of Health and Human Services and its public health agencies on the charge of procrastination in the release of new AIDS therapies, Forrest A. Hainline III, counsel for the plaintiffs, offered the following quote from the preliminary report in support of his contention that NIH was lax in making new AIDS therapies available: "The deadly nature of AIDS demands new and streamlined approaches to drug and vaccine development. . . . The Commission is concerned that after eight years there are so few drug therapies available to AIDS outpatients."

Hainline went on to charge that "NIH has restricted what it will agree to test to two classes of drugs, those developed by its own researchers and those developed by a company with whom it had a close economic relationship." The monopoly position of AZT as the sole authorized AIDS therapy Hainline attributed to "self-dealing and impropriety at NIH and FDA." He noted that upon announcement of the December 16 hearing on the complaint the makers of AZT announced a "probable" 20 percent cut in the price of the drug.

His clients, Hainline declared, were asking the court (even as Cardinal O'Connor had done at the September Commission hearing) "to require the agencies to institute procedures of fairness and accountability so that we know the reasons why a given company's drug is or is not tested and that those reasons [be] articulated and reasonable . . . [and] to require FDA to have a citizen's petition procedure that is adequate for this crisis. Dying people have a right to their bodies and the therapies of their choice."

Hainline's argument was to no avail.

On April 28, 1988 Sherrie Kopka Kennedy, Hainline's associate in the complaint, reported: "On April 26 Judge [Norma Holloway] Johnson granted the government's motion to dismiss NGRA's complaint because of NGRA's failure to exhaust administrative remedies."

◆ ◆ ◆

All was not lost, however, as a result of the dismissal of the NGRA et al. complaint. Unaccustomed to intense and unremitting pressure especially from such a varied opposition—community organizations, state and local officials and Congressional committees—FDA and NIH had earlier sought to mollify their critics. In June 1987, following upon activist demonstrations at the IIIrd International AIDS Conference in Washington and upon the announcement of the NGRA et al. complaint, Anthony Fauci, director of the National Institute of Allergies and Infectious Diseases, assembled an ad hoc committee to review the AIDS Treatment Evaluation Units (ATEUs). In December 1987 the committee issued a report noting serious shortages in staff and funding and a lack of senior leadership and of "a clearly formulated set of policies, procedures, and priorities. So much staff time and effort was required," the report declared, "in developing and implementing clinical protocols that little time was available for correcting weaknesses and improving efficiency and effectiveness of the program itself." The committee suggested the introduction of greater flexibility in organizational structure; criticized the lack of regular communication with the pharmaceutical industry; proposed the creation of advisory committees to review periodically the total program; noted the need for the establishment of specific guidelines for the selection of drugs for clinical trials and of rules for writing, revising, and reviewing protocols; and urged the publication of newsletters to maintain communication with investigators at the ATEUs and with clinical scientists, industry and basic investigators. It called attention to the acute shortage of space in which NIAID conducted its activities. "The 18 staff members currently are housed in 1380 square feet of space. . . . Only one person has a private office, and because of the crowding, there is no way to discuss issues without disturbing others."

The report of Fauci's ad hoc committee proved to be mere window dressing.

At Commission hearings in December 1987 Mathilde Krim offered an outsider's evaluation of the work of the NIAID. She declared that "the business-as-usual review of applications at NIH tak[ing] up to 18 months" during an epidemic that was doubling every twelve to fourteen months was "hardly tolerable." She could not believe that the process could not be reduced to six to eight months. She scored NIAID as having no experience in the organization of large-scale collaborative clinical trials across the country and for taking on "more than it could chew," noting, for example, the failure to involve people outside NIH in designing the AZT trial and to listen to those who complained about the design of the trial. "I think," she concluded, "that the leadership of NIAID is . . . just not . . . up to the challenge."

In April 1988, testifying before the House Subcommittee on Human Resources, Barry Gingell, medical consultant for the Gay Men's Health Crisis and an observer at meetings of the Clinical Trials Advisory Panel, granted that "the AIDS program was significantly restructured as a result of this report . . . and . . . policies and procedures were rewritten. . . . Unfortunately," Gingell noted, "after over four months of operation, little substantive change has occurred in the AIDS program." Decision making rested, he said, with the same people as before; innovation continued to be discouraged; no increase in public disclosure had been instituted regarding drug selection; and protocol development and affected communities still were not permitted any input.[1]

Other spokesmen of the AIDS community were equally as incisive in their criticisms and proposals. Bruce Decker, president of the Health Policy and Research Foundation, an organization based in California, declared to the Commission that bureaucrats and scientists talk of a crisis and yet insist upon conducting business as usual. After the creation of a California FDA the previous month, now through

---

[1] A December 12, 1989, memo from ACT UP/New York to federal agencies and others declared, "After three years supported by hundreds of millions of public funds, the AIDS Clinical Trials Group has yet to develop data leading to a single new treatment for any HIV related condition."

an AIDS Research Tax Credit initiative, California was about to create its own state NIH. Decker recounted specific proposals he had made the previous day to FDA Commissioner Dr. Frank Young: that (1) "in order to create a partnership rather than an adversarial relationship [Young] should meet within . . . thirty days representatives of community and patient groups to get our input and identify prospective subjects for AIDS treatment INDs [for making unavailable drugs available] if premature death is likely without early treatment"; that (2) "the Commissioner appoint a high-ranking [FDA] executive . . . to actively solicit and process on a priority basis AIDS treatment INDs"; and that (3) "the Commissioner seriously consider AIDS treatment INDs from community-based organizations, individual doctors and other nontraditional applicants to demonstrate his commitment to action, not just to high-standing words."

Not confident (on the basis of past experience) that Young would carry out his promise to take action on these proposals, Decker asked the Commission to "request that FDA report back to [the Commission] within 90 days on their progress in the area of these recommendations." (Indeed, Young took no action, but Decker's recommendations, repeated by other witnesses, would be incorporated into the Commission's Final Report.)

Vic Basile, executive director of the Human Rights Campaign Fund, a lesbian and gay Washington lobbying organization, displayed to the Commission two models of medicine cabinets, one "full of bottles to represent the myriad of drugs under investigation as therapies in HIV infection . . . many . . . in widespread, unapproved use in the community"; and the other containing a single bottle, AZT, "the one drug licensed by FDA for the treatment of HIV infection. The contrast," he commented, "represents the tragic chasm between hope and reality for 1.5 million Americans infected with HIV."

In response to a request by Watkins for a memorandum with additional information and proposals, Basile sent the Commission a statement urging that one of the numerous federal agencies supposedly supervising the campaign against the epidemic, the AIDS Executive Task Force, formed in 1984 by Assistant Secretary of HHS Edward Brandt, be entrusted with the role of developing a general strategy for PHS efforts, allocating resources and formulating policies and procedures for informing the public, the Congress and the scientific community about the PHS effort. (The Final Report of the Commission would, indeed, contain a recommendation for a coordinating commission to carry out similar and additional functions.)

The major problem in the treatment IND program, Basile declared, lay not so much with FDA as in "the unwillingness, often for understandable reasons, of companies to apply for treatment INDs." He stressed the need for cooperative agreements under which companies shared information and made drugs available for treatment protocols "in exchange for exclusive marketing rights, technical assistance and other advantages."

The February 1988 Commission hearings on AIDS research, unfortunately, were hampered by the failure of the Commission's staff to invite witnesses from federal agencies, the pharmaceutical industry and AIDS organizations and to include scientists who had publicly criticized the operations of FDA and NIH. In addition, as John James noted in his *AIDS Treatment News*, Commissioners avoided asking pointed questions of witnesses, and considerable self-congratulation, aggrandizement and fluff crept into the testimony. To James, there seemed to have been "a deliberate policy of keeping the witnesses comfortable so they could say more than if they had been on the defensive."

On the other hand, the gentleness of the Commissioners did not deter Martin Delaney of Project Inform from delivering a caustic critique of FDA and NIH manipulation. "I sat here for hours yesterday," said Delaney, speaking out of his extensive experience as an AIDS activist, "listening to testimony [by agency officials] that I felt was vastly removed from the reality that we have experienced in the community. . . . yesterday [we] saw round after round of slick presentations created by public relations specialists and, in fact, they were the same presentations we have heard for the last two years.[2] I have to ask," Delaney continued, "does the Commission seriously believe everything it has heard from the federal agencies over the last two days. . . . It has in effect been asking the fox how things are going on in the chicken house."

Rejecting the official contention that "problems exist primarily as a perception gap between the AIDS community and what in fact has been done for it," Delaney asserted that the spokesmen for the AIDS community who had testified before him and would follow him were "among the 10 or 15 most knowledgeable people in the country on what has been done and how the system actually works. . . . We have followed their procedures, we have tested their systems, we have filled out their paper work, we have repeatedly listened to their same presentations over and over again, and in all honesty . . . we conclude that they are not telling you the whole truth." Despite their self-congratulatory statements, Delaney noted that besides AZT to date FDA had only Trimetrexate as an authorized therapy, and that drug for a few hundred patients suffering from PCP.[3]

---

[2] With presentations prepared in consultation with skillful public relations experts, FDA and NIH officials manipulated all but the most critical and most informed members of their audiences. A few days before the Commission's February hearings at which Delaney testified, in an interview with the *New York Times*, Anthony Fauci gave an example of such FDA–NIH public relations manipulation. According to the *Times*, "Fauci deplored the 'misperception' that 'if we're not testing every conceivable drug in a trial, we're falling short of our responsibility. All too often,' he said, 'some scientist in Europe will throw a chemical into a test tube and report that it inhibits the AIDS virus, or some doctor will report that a patient got better after one treatment.'" With the contempt with which he customarily responded to criticism, he sneered at the AIDS community: "Soon everybody in New York and San Francisco is saying, 'Why aren't you studying this? Thousands of people are dying in the streets, and this at least offers some hope. Why not try it?'" Fauci dismissed such complaints with standard arrogance: "It's not that easy because when scientifically qualified people look closely at such claims, typically, there are no data."

[3] The drug would be available only to patients who had experienced "a severe or life-threatening adverse reaction to approved therapies" and not to those for whom other therapies had merely proved ineffective. "Those patients," noted John James in the March 11 issue of *AIDS Treatment News*, "will be left to die."

After a threat of a lawsuit by Lambda Legal Defense and Education Fund, FDA in the summer

Delaney recalled that from 1981 to 1984 gay activists urged in vain the allocation of "necessary resources to fight this problem"; that in 1982 they had warned of problems in the blood supply, a warning that was ignored; that since 1986 they had been "urging wider trials and investigator-initiated research" and it was not until "yesterday [that you heard] them urge the same thing"; and "since 1984 we have been telling you that there are safe and effective remedies already in use, please listen to us."

L. Patrick Gage, vice president of the multinational firm of Hoffman LaRoche, criticized the NIH for its failure to cooperate effectively with the pharmaceutical industry in the development of new therapies. "Although well-intentioned," he said,

> the NIH controlled ATEUs do not optimally take advantage of the pharmaceutical industry's drug development experience and capability. For example, once a potentially beneficial compound has been discovered in the laboratories of a pharmaceutical company, the primary goal is then to develop and implement the most prompt and efficient clinical plan to determine the efficacy and safety of the drug and to gain approval for marketing. Planning of the clinical development program for the ATEUs involves NIH representatives, extra-mural clinical investigators [and representatives] from the sponsoring company. Complexities of these interactions can lead to delays in making new drugs available. The ATEU attempt to centralize accrual and management of all clinical data from the studies also causes a delay.

Implying that the involvement of NIAID merely complicated the therapy development process, he proposed that pharmaceutical companies "because of their wealth of experience . . . handle data management and be responsible for all elements of a drug development program within their capability while still working within the ATEU program."

(After a visit to FDA headquarters Admiral Watkins expressed astonishment at the fact that FDA had not yet developed software for computerizing the drug approval process!)

Exclusion of Women and Children from Clinical Tests

Why, Herb Spiers of ACT UP asked rhetorically, are "women, blacks, Hispanics, children and drug users somehow innately unqualified for drug trials, for they are woefully underrepresented in trials?" Denise Ribble, a nurse educator at the Community Health Project in New York City and chief spokesman at Commission hearings on the question of the exclusion of women from clinical hearings, also decried a minimalizing of the risk to heterosexual women by an emphasis on transmission

---

of 1988 expanded the Treatment IND program to include all people who did not respond to standard treatment.

to the general population. "Two percent or 2.6 percent transmission in the general population means . . . 226,000 infected women living in New York City right now." In regard to clinical tests, Ribble noted that women were in a double bind: they could not receive experimental drugs because they were excluded from drug trials, and they could not receive drugs now released for compassionate use because the drugs had not been tested on women. Eight years into the epidemic, Denise Ribble noted, scientists still did not know why women infected with HIV became sicker and died faster than men, and there still were no studies addressing co-factor issues in women, although researchers had suggested that "the disease may have a different etiology in women."

A Pediatric Case Study

Exclusion of pediatric AIDS patients from clinical studies provided another complaint of the AIDS community.

Appearing anonymously as "Joe" before the Weiss congressional subcommittee hearings of April 29, 1988, the father of a 2-year-old little girl related a tale of frustration that could be repeated in dozens of cases throughout the nation. Since AZT had not been released for treatment of children with HIV, there was no therapy available to his daughter. Joe's pediatrician was enrolling patients into a study of gamma globulin, but the protocol called for placing 50 percent of the children on a placebo in a double-blind study. "Who had time for a placebo?" Joe exclaimed. "The virus, apparently, was affecting her brain. She stopped talking, she rolled from side to side, her thumbs turned inward, her legs trembled intermittently, she was unable to sit up." The pediatrician called Burroughs Wellcome to request that AZT be released to the child on compassionate leave. Although Joe offered to sign a waiver to release the firm from possible litigation, the request was denied.

Joe called NIH and was told that if his daughter remained alive and a lung infection cleared up, they would accept her in an AZT clinical study. After two weeks or more at NIH, she would return home and continue treatment with a local physician. The NIH answer was tantamount to a rejection. In desperation, Joe appealed to the House subcommittee:

> My daughter and the other infected children need FDA and the federal agencies to speed the development of effective treatment, to release some of these experimental drugs to try to prolong their lives. . . . Let's not sit here and watch our children deteriorate before our eyes. . . . I can tell you that it is a frustrating and horrible sight. It may be too late for my daughter, but maybe for other children out there we can fight a little harder.[4]

---

[4] Although Congress appropriated money in the fall of 1986 for pediatric AIDS trials, the NIAID did not institute pediatric clinical trials until 1988. On October 26, 1989, the Department of Health and Human Services announced that FDA had approved a "treatment IND" application from Burroughs Wellcome, allowing the company to distribute the drug free for children who met certain medical requirements. AZT had already been given to at least 200 children in clinical trials; it seemed to be no more or less toxic to them than to adults, and it seemed clearly beneficial in some cases.

The Treatment IND

A critical issue in the December and February Commission hearings was the treatment IND regulation promulgated in June 1987 for accelerating the process of making unauthorized therapies available to patients in a life-threatening stage of HIV infection.

To the official claim that there were "no statutory obstacles preventing access to helpful drugs," Delaney responded, "We . . . have experienced a system in which we are denied access to dozens of drugs which have shown promise in early trials." To the claim that "drugs may be made available on the basis of many possible criteria," Delaney countered, "We have experienced a system which has denied treatment IND for drugs which have met all of those criteria." Regarding official claims for success of the treatment IND program, Delaney commented, "We have experienced a system which has delivered a single drug." Of the official assurances of "new treatment INDS coming just around the corner," Delaney remarked, "We have heard that same promise virtually every month for the last year and have not seen the results."

Jay Lipner, a legal counsel for the New York Gay Men's Health Crisis and himself an ARC patient, called the Commission's attention to a list appearing in the January 19, 1988 issue of "Update," a publication of the pharmaceutical manufacturers association, of "all the anti-virals and of all the immunomodulators presently under FDA trials [a total of eighteen drugs]. Under FDA's set of regulations," he noted, these would be likely candidates for treatment INDs. He said:

> People with full-blown AIDS do not have the time to wait until clinical trials have been completed to find out what other drugs are fully effective. . . . If you use that standard, the regulations are meaningless . . . and the treatment IND regulation . . . is going to serve what it has served so far . . . basically an opportunity for FDA to get good press and to create the impression that it is making progress in the battle against AIDS. . . . as we sit here discussing this issue, the situation remains as it was on May 22, 1987, when the regulations were issued.

The French Example

At the first Commission hearings in September 1987 Congressman Ted Weiss charged that in its public education program "the United States . . . lags far behind countries like Great Britain, Denmark, Switzerland and Australia, which have far fewer people with AIDS or HIV infection." Two months later, Dr. Roy Widdus, director of the Institute of Medicine of the Academy of Sciences, urged the Commission to look at the experiences of certain European nations and of Australia for lessons for the U.S. approach to the AIDS crisis. At Commission hearings in February 1988, decrying the "lackadaisical political and medical response" in the United States to the epidemic during the first years of its spread, Dr. Herb Spiers of ACT UP urged creation of an ombuds agency "to examine the experience of other countries in the search for new drugs."

In April 1988 the Commission had the opportunity to investigate the French response to the AIDS crisis upon the testimony of Alain Pompidou, technical counsel for health of the Ministry of Health and the Family and head of the French program.

In introducing Pompidou, Commissioner Walsh declared: "I was very much impressed when I was last in France to find how the government of France was already well to the forefront of attempting to help many countries in the Third World, while at the same time devoting attention to solving the problems of AIDS in their own country and actually in providing leadership for a good part of Western Europe."

In a cogent, detailed description of the French mobilization against the epidemic, Pompidou described a national committee of scientists, ethicists and health educators as well as representatives of the arts, pharmaceutical firms, insurance companies and the clergy, who served as an advisory board to the ministry. A national coordinator, he declared, ensured coordination among the various ministries and bore responsibility for international collaborative efforts and for maintaining contact with private groups, including foundations and industry as well as gay organizations.

The French AIDS program had two components: (1) prevention, including education (directed toward both the general public and health service providers) and screening; and (2) research, health services and international cooperation. Mandatory testing had been instituted for blood and organ donors. A hundred centers provided free and anonymous testing, and in 1986 800,000 and in 1987 2.4 million blood donors voluntarily submitted to testing. Betrayal of confidentiality could result in loss of a physician's license.

Twenty-two pilot centers provided care facilities, each associated with a network of regional hospitals. Research was coordinated by the Ministry for Research and Universities. In the spring of 1988 more than fifty research teams were working on HIV infection studies or on socio-economic aspects of the disease.

Medical contact had been established with about half the IV drug users in the country, and one-third of these were enrolled in detoxification centers. The national rate of HIV infection among drug abusers ranged from 40 percent to as high as 80 percent in Marseilles. Syringes were available without prescription in pharmacies. The sale of condoms increased almost 40 percent in one year.

Although, indeed, major differences existed in the AIDS crisis in the two nations—France had fewer AIDS cases than any of the American cities with major concentrations; it is a smaller, compact, comparatively homogeneous nation with a tradition of political centralization—it was clear from Pompidou's report that much could be learned from the French experience. Members of the Commission, however, posed no questions of substance to their French guest. Pompidou seemed to have been invited to testify to no greater purpose than to provide the Commission with an interesting afternoon.

Questioned subsequently about this failure to take advantage of a unique opportunity, Admiral Watkins explained that he had had to miss the session at which Pompidou spoke. "I would have known," he said, "how to elicit the kind of information that would have been useful for a comparison of national efforts. The French do begin with a certain rationality that we lack."

Hearings of House and Senate Committees

At hearings on April 28 and 29, 1988, complementing the investigations of the Presidential Commission and, indeed, in collaboration with the Commission's staff, the House Subcommittee on Human Services sought to evaluate the progress of FDA and NIH in developing new therapies. (Proposals and criticisms at these hearings would be included in the Commission's Final Report.) Representatives of the AIDS community once again provided astute testimony.

Mathilde Krim offered specific recommendations for the acceleration of the review of AIDS-related grant proposals, for funding at the 50 percent level of approved applications without a delay of six months from the date of receipt of an application, for creating or enlarging training grants for the expert manpower required to deal with the epidemic, for encouraging industrial companies to participate in clinical research and for clarifying for the medical community both the drugs available as compassionate IND drugs and the implications of the treatment IND.

Kevin Armington of the Gay Men's Health Crisis of New York, appearing in place of ailing PWA Barry Gingell, described the community advisory board created in San Francisco to meet with the local ATEU as "a model that should exist on a national scale." He urged the creation of an official organism to call regular meetings between groups in the AIDS community and FDA and NIH for the exchange of views and for checking on the implementation of suggestions.

David Barr, a staff attorney of the gay defense organization Lambda Legal Defense and Education Fund, charged that FDA had issued such conflicting messages about standards in determining treatment IND application approval that drug companies and researchers were reluctant to seek treatment IND status for their products. Barr noted a particular weakness in the treatment IND regulation: the decision to apply for treatment IND status for a product depended solely upon the manufacturer, who could block such action and prevent his product from reaching individuals who might benefit from it.

Dr. Iris Long, a pharmaceutical physicist and a member of the Issues Committee of ACT UP and the data section of its Treatment and Data Subcommittee, told the House subcommittee that people infected with HIV had become so distrustful of placebo trials that a clinical test of AZT for AIDS dementia complex had succeeded in enrolling only 34 patients instead of the 315 mandated in the protocol. Researchers in the study, Dr. Long declared, treated patients as mere objects of a clinical project. A member of ACT UP, she reported, was kept in the dark regarding his diagnosis and intimidated when he asked questions. For sixteen weeks, he said, patients were given no medication against depression or to alleviate the pain of monthly spinal taps.

As an example of the disarray in the official research program, Dr. Long pointed to the absence of a registry of government or private treatment trial information. To fill the need for such data, the treatment subcommittee of ACT UP, of which she was chairman, was developing an electronic registry of clinical trials in the New York area.

Admiral Watkins summarized much of what he had learned from the several hundred witnesses before the Commission and from investigations conducted by the Commission's staff. "The nation," Watkins charged, "was not ready to deal with a new infectious disease. . . . In fact, we as a nation have become so chronically self-satisfied in our technological achievements in the health area that we have been lulled into woeful unpreparedness to deal with a new virus. . . . after seven years into this medical crisis our bureaucracy is still trying to struggle out of its lethargy."

Anthony Fauci on the Stand

Subcommittee Chairman Ted Weiss of New York and committee members Nancy Pelosi and Henry A. Waxman of California—all three from districts with major concentrations of HIV infection—had had much experience over more than five years in questioning officials of government agencies responsible for the struggle against the AIDS epidemic. At the April 1988 hearings, with undisguised impatience they pressed NIAID director Fauci for an explanation for the current authorization of only a single AIDS therapy.

Unable to silence criticism from these experienced investigators by standard pat phrases, Fauci pleaded a shortage of personnel. "We requested 127 FTEs [full-time employees] and received this past year 11. . . . the amount that was gotten at the Department [of Health and Human Services] was less than was asked for."

Dr. Jack Killen, an associate of Fauci's, later admitted in a telephone conversation with a member of ACT UP that NIAID had actually received only five additional full-time staff people. Fauci, a loyal administration man, did not disclose that fact to the subcommittee.

When Waxman asked about the failure to institute pediatric trials, Fauci waffled. "I think it is an important problem," he said, "and right now we're not doing as much as we'd like to do, and we're going to improve that." Charged by Weiss with having accomplished very little in drug development, Fauci admitted: "If you think in terms of the concept of a cure and having drugs that are available for everyone, relatively speaking what has been accomplished is very little."

Weiss asked Fauci whether in fiscal 1989 he needed $30 million above the president's budget request for his clinical research units. Cautious of criticizing the Reagan administration, Fauci replied that ATEU investigators submitted their estimates only after the publication of the president's budget. He had no reason to believe, however, that Weiss's figure of an additional $30 million needed for clinical research units was incorrect. Fauci also admitted that because of a shortage in appropriations there had been "some diminution in training" of AIDS researchers for future needs. (Less than three months later, Fauci would about-face and assure presidential candidate George Bush that no additional funds were needed for AIDS research!)

Noting that under the newly established California State Drug Administration, "a drug is brought forth and within a week it is messengered all over the state, a committee is formed immediately," Pelosi asked whether there was not some way to accelerate the national drug trial program in a similar fashion. The process, Fauci responded, was going "much faster" and he and his colleagues were "trying to look for ways to expedite in a more intensive fashion."

When Weiss noted that the clinical trials programs were hampered by a shortage of facilities, Fauci outdid himself in his mastery of bureaucratese. "There's no question," he said, "that it has a negative effect both on the research itself and on the safety." Funds had been received "for infrastructure in NIH to expand the facilities at NCI and NIAID."

Questioned regarding action to prevent the exorbitant prices of AIDS therapies, Fauci replied with more bureaucratese: "Due to the fact that it became clear that certain drugs were very expensive and in certain cases out of the reach of people who needed the drugs the most, there is a pattern now being established at NIH that when NIH engages in a cooperative agreement whereby we would have a patent for the drug and grant exclusive licensure to a given drug company with a proviso that we would have say in the keeping the price of that drug reasonable."

Turning to Dr. Daniel Hoth, an associate of Fauci, Weiss noted the absence of IVDUs, women, children and people of color from clinical trials. Hoth replied in equally well-practiced bureaucratese: "We have no policy which excludes any group. What we are looking at now is a generation of a more proactive policy to study these other important groups."

Peggy Dufour, a senior staff member on the Presidential Commission and a friend of Fauci and Fauci's family, attempted to explain Fauci's fudging on fundamental questions. Upon arriving in Washington, she had been dismayed to discover that top-level officials in the Department of Health and Human Services were hardly concerned about anything but holding the line on the budget. "People on the second level," she declared, "were different. . . . working ten-hour days seven days a week . . . individuals like Tony Fauci. If only Dr. Fauci could do what he wanted to do!" she exclaimed. "There are four or five layers above him, and then there's OMB" (the Office of Management and Budget).

How did Dufour account for the fact that Fauci's public statements did not bear out her characterization of him? "When he gives irrational responses," Dufour replied:

> Tony's job as a spokesman is to say what the Administration wants him to say.
> He has gone farther than anyone in the opposite direction in actually saying,
> "These are the numbers that we asked for and the word came back . . . what we
> could officially ask for." He could lose his job for saying that. He has a real fear.
> His family is afraid. . . . Seeing these people who you expect to be advocates
> have to play this dual role is the worst thing we could have in a situation
> like this.

Commissioner Young on the Stand

To Congressman Weiss's question whether "the staffing and funding levels requested [by FDA] for fiscal year 1989 [would] be adequate for the AIDS work load," Young admitted that because of fiscal restraints FDA had had to "reduce . . . efforts in a number of fields." Recently, thirty additional staff people had been hired, but there was no space in FDA headquarters to put them.

When Pelosi asked Young whether he would use unauthorized therapies if he were infected with HIV, Young replied, "I would take the best treatments that I thought were available." For that reason, he said, FDA had adopted a policy under which "we have not defied [sic] individuals . . . from the seeking of medicines from underground clinics."

Noting that a year earlier he had been criticized for "not requiring enough efficacy on the treatment IND," now, Young said, "I would be delighted to go back and review this." (The committee members had heard such promises before and were apparently too weary to comment on this remark.)

Frustrated with remarks by both Young and his assistant Dr. Ellen Cooper, Pelosi exclaimed, "I've heard comments today about limited data, limited drugs, limited patients, no methodology. . . . What I can see about the treatment INDs is a lot more promise than real product."

Young claimed a 50 percent achievement. He had, after all, approved one of two drugs for which application had been made!

Criticism of the treatment IND continued at July hearings of the Senate Committee on Labor and Human Resources. Dr. John F. Bear, senior vice president for science and technology of the Pharmaceutical Manufacturers Association, declared that "in a situation now where there are a million to 1.5 million people infected with the virus, it is difficult to see how the primary care doctors . . . are going to be able to cope with complex procedures to obtain medications . . . in the context of a busy practice where the beeper is going off and there is one patient on the phone and one sitting in front of you and a third ailing and with only months to live."

Speaking as the medical consultant for the Gay Men's Health Crisis of New York and as a Person with AIDS, Barry Gingell charged the institution of the treatment IND had "falsely and cruelly raised the hopes of people with AIDS. . . . It is no act of kindness," he said, "to tell us that help is on the way when the reality is that nothing has changed at all."

Gingell went on to deliver a pungent rejoinder to the standard presentations by both Fauci and Young, a comprehensive exposé of years of empty verbiage and arrogant, self-serving rationalizations for bureaucratic incompetence. The AIDS drug development program, Gingell characterized as

> a brand new Government bureaucracy with an annual budget approaching $150 million that has: one, put most of its eggs in one basket—that is, AZT; two, spent 2 years reinventing certain systems that exist in abundance in the private sector; and, three, exerted most of its energy endlessly scrutinizing new ideas instead of rapidly investing resources in those ideas to get desperately needed answers.
>
> I advocate . . . an overall approach to AIDS drug evaluation that is consistent with the urgency of the epidemic. . . . The whole point of assembling this enormous network of medical institutions called the AIDS clinical trial

group is to be able to get a well-designed clinical trial up and rolling rapidly, to have qualified investigators at multiple centers working to find answers on toxicity and efficacy on as many promising agents as possible. Unfortunately, to date, that just is not happening.

Gingell countered, one by one, standard rationalizations advanced by Fauci and his colleagues: "We must do nothing that could harm patients. . . . These things just take time." "In fact," commented Gingell, "there has not been a drug in history that did not entail a margin of risk to early recipients. Calculating what is an 'acceptable' margin of risk depends on the threat posed by the illness. . . . we are a long way from the point at which our experimental treatment efforts . . . could be said to constitute a greater hazard to HIV-infected people than HIV itself."

In response to the Establishment argument that "it is better to focus our energies on the few drugs that are really promising," Gingell asked:

> How do we find out what is actually promising without doing studies? The only reliable test of what works must be carried out in people. We have not even started the work that must be done to find out which of many candidate therapies is most promising. Apart from a few studies to gain a better understanding of AZT, Dr. Fauci seems to be telling us that the NIH AIDS drug program has spent most of the last two years getting staffed and organized.

A third argument, "We only have so much money and cannot pursue every drug that comes along," Gingell rejected by exclaiming, "I do not know what more the United States Congress can do to demonstrate its willingness to spend what is needed to put the AIDS nightmare behind us."

Seeking to blunt the mounting criticism against his agency, on July 23, 1988, in Boston in an address at the Lesbian and Gay Health Conference, Young announced that FDA would permit patients to import up to a three-month supply of unapproved medicines for personal use. (Martin Delaney had negotiated this concession with the Commissioner specifically in regard to Dextran sulfate, a new AIDS drug that was being imported from Japan, Mexico and Canada by hundreds of individuals with HIV infection.)

John James commented in *AIDS Treatment News* on July 28:

> If FDA's new announcement proves effective in practice, it will let everyone focus less on fights over access and more on how we can work together to get treatments tested and made available. . . . And legal access to drugs not yet approved in this country could end the festering scandal of drugs used by thousands of people in Europe, Japan, or elsewhere being unavailable to Americans. . . . In the past these drugs have been accessible only to those Americans who could afford to travel to pick them up.

Mid-Level Blockage at FDA

On January 17, 1989, at a meeting of a group of San Francisco PWAs afflicted with CMV retinitis, an opportunistic eye disease that can lead to blindness, Delaney discussed with Fauci the possibility of a reversal of an FDA demand for further testing of gamcyclovir, a drug that was widely prescribed by physicians as an effective cure for the disease.

Acknowledging that plenty of experience on hand demonstrated the effectiveness of the drug, Fauci disagreed with FDA on its refusal to permit use of gamcyclovir without requiring the standard testing procedure, which might delay use of the drug for years. He was prepared, he said, to make such a statement before a congressional committee if called upon.

Delaney noted that the problem was going to be Ellen Cooper and the mid-level staff at FDA. Fauci responded, "I know."

(Fauci's willingness to support Delaney in requesting FDA action on gamcyclovir represented a turnaround for him. Confident as newly appointed AIDS adviser to president-elect Bush, Fauci now dared to express forthright and unequivocal opinions instead of the obfuscating bureaucratese that he had employed previously.)

ELLEN COOPER, THE GATEKEEPER

The *New York Times*, briefed by ACT UP, carried a story of Fauci's subsequent appeal to Frank Young regarding gamcyclovir and of Young's agreement to reconsider the FDA decision to demand clinical trials before releasing the drug. When Jay Lipner, representing Project Inform, mentioned the report to Cooper, she replied, "Don't believe everything you read in the papers."

Some months later, after Cooper had delivered a standard FDA public relations speech at a meeting of the San Francisco County Community Consortium, Delaney and several other AIDS activists questioned her on the contradiction between Commissioner Young's promise, frequently repeated, of patient access under the treatment IND regulation to promising drugs that had not undergone the required clinical trials and the actuality under which FDA insisted upon proof of effectiveness before releasing therapies for terminal cases of HIV infection.

"I don't care what the Commissioner says," responded Cooper. "I wish he wouldn't say those things. We all groan when he speaks on this subject."

(At a meeting of the Institute of Medicine Roundtable on February 18, 1989 Young complained of being obstructed by the middle management of his agency. He did not have a free hand, he admitted, in developing policy. He suggested that scientific committees of unimpeachable credentials present reports on individual drugs for him to use in compelling action from his subordinates.)

On August 19, 1988, in an article headed "Food and Drug Administration: At Fulcrum of Conflict, Regulator of AIDS Drugs," the *New York Times* characterized Cooper "as the most important gatekeeper for AIDS drugs in the nation, a role that has caught her in a spotlight of conflict that is rare for someone who is a mid-level manager at the Food and Drug Administration." After noting that Cooper had been praised for expediting the authorization of AZT, the *Times* article went on to say that "to her critics among organizations that serve AIDS patients, she is cold, heartless, inexperienced and so determined to follow the strict scientific process that she needlessly denies dying patients drugs whose value has not been fully proven, though the patients are willing and eager to try them."[5]

◆ ◆ ◆

Dubious of Cooper's qualifications upon first meeting her in July 1987, Delaney requested a copy of her curriculum vitae. His request was denied.

In mid-April 1988 a Freedom of Information request for the curricula vitae for both Cooper and her associate Nazim Moledina was submitted for this book. Acknowledgment of the request arrived six weeks later. At the end of June, in a telephone conversation, Gerald Deighton, director of the Freedom of Information staff of FDA, promised that a reply would be forthcoming within a week. A threat of an appeal for the intervention of Congressman Ted Weiss at the end of July brought a response in August, four months after the original request, in regard to Cooper. For Moledina, Deighton declared no curriculum was available. He advised the submission of a further request for a copy of Moledina's employment application form.

A request was filed in mid-August. Acknowledgment of the request arrived on August 29.

The request was denied in September.

Further correspondence, including an appeal of the denial, followed during October and November.

On January 6, 1989, nine months after the initial request, FDA provided a copy of Molidena's curriculum vitae (in contradiction to the previous declaration that no curriculum vitae existed for her).

Sent the documents for evaluation, Delaney commented regarding the Cooper curriculum: "I saw nothing in there that qualifies her as a top level researcher or suggests that she is in a position to judge top level researchers." Of the Moledina document, he declared:

> I'm even more dismayed than I expected to be. I don't see anything there that remotely qualifies that woman for this position. Her background, a small background, is in pediatrics. She has no research experience, no statistical experience, no virology experience. A few years as a physician in pediatrics and a couple of years in a fellowship in infectious diseases. The document is entitled CV. Actually it is a fairly crude resume. She has never been published. You can understand why they were reluctant to send it.

---

[5] At the April 1988 hearings of the Weiss House subcommittee, Lambda Legal Defense and Education Fund attorney David Barr reported that at a meeting with Young and a number of FDA officials, "Dr. Cooper said to me that she felt that she was wasting her time by meeting with people like me."

"The only thing the two women are qualified for," Delaney observed, "is to carry on the tradition of the agency, to carry out the regulations according to the book, as they were trained to do upon being hired. I don't see them bringing anything new or any scientific expertise." Regarding the two women, Delaney quoted a leading San Francisco AIDS researcher, Dr. Vera Byers: "People who are judging our work are people who failed in qualifying or have no qualifications at all."

Increasingly beleaguered by AIDS community criticism, Cooper agreed to meet with AIDS activists in San Francisco on February 16, 1989, but on condition that they not invite anybody who would shout at her. "ACT UP," explained Delaney, "has been zapping her and she's become teary."

At the meeting Cooper insisted that the data in support of gamcyclovir (DHPG) supplied by Syntex, the manufacturer (which had supplied 2,700 patients with the drug at no cost on a compassionate use protocol), had been too spotty and impressionistic to enable the FDA advisory panel in October 1987 to hand down any other ruling than to require clinical tests. (Experience had shown, in fact, that 80 percent of PWAs afflicted with CMV retinitis treated with the drug did not lose their sight, while 100 percent of those not treated with the drug did become blind.) The vote of the panel had been eleven to two, with the two ophthalmologists holding out for a favorable recommendation.

Dr. Iris Long, who attended the panel hearing on the drug, presented an account of the October 1987 proceedings of the advisory panel to the Treatment and Data Committee of ACT UP, and the committee began an investigation of the drug.

When on November 30, 1988 FDA announced a four-tiered set of protocols for testing gamcyclovir, an ACT UP group met with ophthalmologists who had experience with the drug and found universal agreement that the drug worked. A *New York Times* correspondent investigated the ACT UP charge that "FDA and NIH were playing games with the sight of people with AIDS," and on February 1, 1988 thirty members of ACT UP traveled to a Washington meeting of the National Committee to Review Current Procedures for Approval of New Drugs for Cancer and AIDS at which the drug was to be discussed. "We were angry at [Cooper]," reported Bill Bahlman, "because she and other representatives of FDA . . . were in a position to approve DHPG but chose not to. It was not their eyesight that was at risk." When Cooper rose to speak, the ACT UP people held up some twenty-five posters with the slogans: "See the Light, DHPG Works" and "FDA Is Making People with AIDS Go Blind."

In her remarks Cooper repeated the stale story of the rapid approval of AZT but made no mention of DHPG. When she finished speaking, the ACT UP people shouted, "What about DHPG?" Cooper returned to the podium and read a prepared statement. She faced severe questioning from the ACT UP members but refused to change her position.

Later that day Fauci agreed to meet with three representatives of ACT UP in Bethesda. He promised to urge Commissioner Young to reexamine the data on DHPG.

Thus when Martin Delaney, unaware of the ACT UP actions two weeks earlier, warned Cooper that if FDA deprived patients of a drug of generally recognized effectiveness, the AIDS community would mount a powerful attack on the agency, Cooper, already intimidated, retreated. A way had to be found, she said, to permit the prescription of gamcyclovir immediately, without, however, establishing a precedent for ignoring FDA regulations in the future. She asked Delaney's assistance.

(For the AIDS community a precedent regarding the necessity for adapting regulations in a situation of crisis was desirable. FDA could not be permitted to continue its time-consuming procedures with AIDS therapies as it might do, for example, with treatments for athlete's foot.)

On May 2, 1988, at a reconvening of the Committee to Review Procedures, Cooper, Bill Bahlman reported, "began the session by saying that she could not think of a single reason why the committee should not move to recommend approval of DHPG." The committee voted with a single abstention in favor of approval. (FDA, however, did not grant approval of DHPG until a year later.)

"Who wants to serve at FDA?" asked Admiral Watkins. "The very best people should be there. . . . Now they lose their best people to the pharmaceutical industry. They bring in some lesser light to judge somebody they consider better qualified. The situation is backwards."

The Office of Management and Budget

During the Reagan administration, OMB (a White House agency) served as a watchdog over funding for domestic programs. Repeatedly it cut appropriation requests of the Department of Health and Human Services and its dependent agencies. During July 1988 hearings of the Senate Committee on Labor and Human Resources, Commission member Dr. Burton Lee graphically exposed its high-handed interventions. Lee testified that many of the people at NIH "told us about how the budget proposals, the personnel proposals, have to carry up through the Public Health Service, HHS, OMB and come back. . . . the director [of NIH] has lost control of his organization. We [the Presidential Commission] are recommending . . . that NIH be cut loose . . . and that [its budget] not be micromanaged by OMB." According to Lee, OMB played a numbers game with national health research. "A total of 371 [full-time employees] were [approved] for HIV, but [NIH] lost overall 1,032. . . . this is OMB telling Wyngaarden . . . that he is going to lose so many positions in cancer and heart disease, mental disease, etc. . . . If these cutbacks were being made by the director, as a commission we can understand. We don't understand that this type of cutback is made by OMB."

To Watkins's complaint that "OMB was not very receptive to our commission when we went over to find out what was going on. . . . it seems to me they sit there making judgments as a surrogate secretary for medical research . . . without portfolio," Senator Lowell Weicker responded:

The question has been asked each of the last four years who OMB has on their staff passing upon this budget that has medical qualifications or scientific qualifications . . . the answer . . . is none, zero. . . . Not only have you been given a hard time as a commission, but so has the entire Congress of the United States, and therefore, the people of the United States, by a group that has absolutely no qualifications at all, either to set the totals or to manage.

The Community Research Initiative

"A lot of people are very much of the belief that what the doctor says, you do," Tom Jefferson told the *Los Angeles Times* on August 16, 1987. (Director of the hotline for Project Inform and organizer with John Fox of the San Francisco Healing Alternatives, Tom enjoyed the respect of PWA activists throughout the United States.) On the other hand, a change of attitude, Tom declared, was taking place, "particularly with people who have been affected by the AIDS virus. I've never felt that MD stood for 'medal of deity.'"

Ironically, Tom himself was to provide an example of the danger of exaggerated trust in physicians. In October 1987 at the Veterans Administration hospital in San Diego researchers involved in an AIDS Test Evaluation Unit clinical study put Tom on Fansidar, an experimental drug, without warning him of possible dangerous side effects. In less than a week, Tom came down with Stevens-Johnson's disease. "Over the next two weeks," reported Martin Delaney in a eulogy published in *AIDS Treatment News*, "this led to treatment with massive doses of Prednisone, which shut the rash down, and his entire immune system along with it." Tom developed pneumonia and legionnaires' disease. After a week in a respirator, Tom, too weary to continue to fight, left the hospital to spend Christmas with his family. He died the day after Christmas.

"It is a great irony," commented Delaney, "that after successfully managing his own illness, Tom finally succumbed not to HIV but to complications of treatment with a drug he was forced to use against his will. . . . The real story of his death is one of bureaucratic obstinacy and competitive behavior between researchers."

Subsequently, over a period of three months, Project Inform received reports of three deaths caused by Fansidar. "Yet," declared Delaney, "it is given to gay men with deeply compromised health despite the availability of better and safer treatments." Delaney concluded: "Tom's experience can't help but make us wonder how many of our brothers' deaths, attributed to HIV, really occurred when a patient was caught in a whirlpool of causes and effects set off by one false move, one bureaucratic stall, one act of ego or medical arrogance. How much does the life expectancy of AIDS patients depend upon where and from whom they are getting their treatment?"

While FDA and NIH dallied and engaged in self-serving publicity campaigns, PWAs took action in developing a program of their own for testing new therapies. In New York the Community Research Initiative (CRI), established at the initiative in 1986 of the Persons with AIDS Coalition, by the spring of 1987 had assembled forty of the most experienced and dedicated AIDS physicians in the city to undertake large-scale, coordinated drug trials at the level of the primary care provider.[6]

By the fall of 1987 a board of governors was meeting weekly, and a Scientific Advisory Committee had been formed to generate and review ideas for research. With an Institutional Review Board (IRB) approved by New York State and empowered to oversee clinical trials, the CRI set to organizing testing through local community physicians, many of whom were associated with leading hospitals and research centers. PWAs, including women, minorities and IVDUs—groups overlooked by NIH—participated as partners in the clinical trials.

Following a more compassionate approach than NIH, CRI designed studies without the use of placebos so that no group of patients would be sacrificed for the sake of "saving" a test. In developing protocols, CRI researchers took into consideration the reality that their patients were taking other substances.

Testifying before the Presidential Commission, Dr. Krim explained that with any therapy for this disease experimental, research effort had to be expanded quickly. Such efforts did not necessarily require large sums or special sophistication in some areas. "Even at the community level in the hands of community physicians," she insisted, "a lot of useful work can be done, useful from the standpoint of the patient and useful from the standpoint of research."

In September CRI received a $51,000 contribution from a Long Island group called People Taking Action against AIDS for a large-scale clinical test of the egg lecithin variant AL721 to be conducted under Sonnabend's direction. The PWA Health Group, thriving as a distributor of AL721 analogs, donated $1,401 toward CRI rent and the purchase of a copying machine.

Negotiations were begun with Dupont and HMR Medical Research Co. for a $3–4 million study of Ampligen involving 200 PWAs. "Although it is a placebo-controlled study," the CRI interim report of September 29, 1987 noted, "the pharmaceutical company would be willing to incorporate the design provisions suggested by Dr. Sonnabend and the IRB protecting the placebo-control group with prophylaxis for PCP for all participants and an unblinding of the study in the event of any decline of the condition of any patient."

A protocol was submitted to the CRI Investigational Review Board by Ortho Pharmaceutical Corporation for a study to be directed by CRI physician Barbara

---

6 Community-based AIDS research in New York dates to 1983, when Drs. Joseph Sonnabend and Mathilde Krim founded the AIDS Medical Foundation to initiate clinical trials in collaboration with local physicians who were providing care to gay men. The foundation's first trial, on the effects of isoprinosine, was conducted in the office of Dr. Joyce Wallace. In 1985 the AIDS Medical Foundation joined with a California group to establish American Foundation for AIDS Research (AmFAR). AmFAR shifted its focus to laboratory research in place of community-based research. In the summer of 1989 AmFAR established the Community-Based Clinical Trials Network (CBCT) under whose auspices representatives of working groups meet regularly. AmFAR also extended emergency funding to twelve local research groups.

Starett of its product Recombinant Human Erythropoietin, a therapy for anemia caused either by HIV or as a result of the use of AZT.

CRI physician Jeffrey Ashkenazi of Montefiore Hospital obtained funding from NIH and from the Baxter-Travenoll Corp., manufacturer of Intralipid 20—a lipid with a proportion of components different from AL721—for a study involving the implantation of a catheter with the substance into PWAs suffering from malnutrition. (With these funds Ashkenazi was able to assign a woman on his staff to work at CRI headquarters.) The CRI IRB was planning to submit a formal protocol to FDA for a dose-ranging study.

In October CRI negotiated a $300,000 contract with LyphoMed for a 200-patient study of aerosolized pentamidine, a prophylaxis against PCP. The study, in fulfillment of a phase of required FDA testing, would be accomplished by CRI at minimal cost and without the bureaucratic complications to be met elsewhere. A further trial involving LyphoMed and Fizons Corporation would test the drug with 500 PWARCs.

Bristol Myers sponsored a CRI study of a therapy for cryptosporidiosis, a devastating opportunistic diarrhea. Plans were drafted for the Lange Project, named for the initiator Dr. Michael Lange of St. Luke's/Roosevelt Medical Center, to assemble information from the thousands of patients treating themselves with unauthorized therapies.

CRI projected the development of a computerized database of treatment information for rapid transmission to physicians and for reviewing results of research efforts throughout the nation. In testimony before the Presidential Commission on February 19, 1988 Tom Hannan, acting director of CRI, declared: "Although there is precedence for community sponsored research, the most exciting aspect of this project is that it originates from the AIDS community, empowering ourselves to participate in the research that may save our lives and dramatically expand the number of patients who have access to experimental drugs."

Michael Callen told the Commission: "We keep hearing [from Fauci] that there are all these problems in starting and designing clinical trials. . . . In six months we have approved 5 trials, 3 of which are already enrolling patients. So it can be done. . . . What seems to be lacking [at NIH] is sufficient political will."

The December 1987 report of the AIDS Clinical Trials Advisory Group set up by Anthony Fauci urged the exploration of "innovative opportunities for community-based providers to perform clinical research . . . [to] permit more rapid completion of certain types of clinical trials, accelerate the transfer of new therapies from research to practice, and provide alternative sources of information for participating physicians," and in September 1987 an AIDS projects coordinator, Dr. Daniel Hoth, was appointed at NIH as director for clinical studies.

At Commission hearings, addressing Hannan, Dr. Lee quoted Hoth as testifying on the previous day that he was "strongly on your side. I would hope," said Lee, "in the next six months I would hear more cooperation from your end instead of this constant bashing [of NIH and FDA]." Tom Hannan replied that he had sought contact with Hoth six months earlier. He hoped that the collaboration promised by Hoth could be accomplished soon.[7]

Two of the Commissioners praised the CRI effort from their own conservative point of view. John Creedon, chief executive officer of Metropolitan Life, observed: "What you are doing is introducing an element of competition into the realm of ideas on how to deal with the AIDS problem." He suggested that CRI consider applying to the insurance industry for help.

Dr. Walsh, too, expressed his enthusiasm. He noted the problems pharmaceutical companies were encountering with the ATEUs. He was sure that the CRI method of clinical trials was closer to what pharmaceutical companies normally did in clinical trials. "Let us know," he urged Hannan, "specifically . . . what we can do to get more support . . . directed to community-based trials, modeled after your experience."

Admiral Watkins described CRI as "at the heart of a concept . . . that needs to be critically looked at [in] a rapidly moving emerging crisis." He called CRI a "tremendous adjunct to what can and should be done at the national level." Hannan assured the Commissioners that CRI sought to encourage other communities to develop similar programs, to the point of preparing how-to packets.

Appearing before the Weiss subcommittee in April 1988, Hannan expressed the demands of PWAs regarding research, insisting that it "proceed expeditiously and properly, that it exhaust every lead. We have a responsibility to those we have allowed to die, like my lover [Steve Roach], who died in my arms in January. And we have a responsibility to those that still have a chance to live."

(After lingering with deteriorating health for more than a year, Tom Hannan died in June 1991.)

Callen expressed a sentiment of many in the AIDS community when he declared to the Presidential Commission that apart from CRI he saw "no other creative solutions to the logjam in the federal treatment research." He called for creation of a treatments Manhattan Project that would pursue every reasonable lead with all due haste.

The only effort in the nation similar to CRI's was San Francisco's County Community Consortium, established in 1985 to facilitate communication between local physicians and the AIDS staff at San Francisco General Hospital. In an interview for *AIDS Treatment News*, Dr. Donald Abrams of the hospital and chairman of the consortium characterized CRI in New York as "a little more aggressive in trying to obtain drugs for early private-practice trials," activity beyond the capacities of the San Francisco group. On the other hand, in July 1987, upon reports of success in New York with aerosolized pentamidine, 440 patients were enrolled in a cooperative San Francisco study.

---

[7] Almost a year and a half later, in the fall of 1989, NIAID at last established Community Programs for Clinical Research on AIDS with a budget of $9 million to fund community-based groups. Of the four New York groups funded by the new agency, none expected to begin clinical trials in 1990.

In July 1988 AmFAR awarded $30,000 to CRI and $50,427 to the County Community Consortium for testing AIDS treatments through patient volunteers in physicians' private practices.

The Community Research Alliance (CRA)

In the fall of 1988 CRA was established in San Francisco, modeled on New York's Community Research Initiative and, like CRI, sponsored by the local PWA Coalition. Five San Francisco AIDS groups each contributed $1,000 to fund the new organization. In the December 1, 1988 issue of *AIDS Treatment News*, John James, one of the founders of CRA, explained that because the County Community Consortium was able to conduct only a limited number of trials at a time and did not involve PWAs in policymaking, organization and administration, San Francisco required another organization.

According to James:

> Pharmaceutical companies are only likely to support products which will provide them with the highest return. . . . It is no coincidence that AZT, one of the most expensive drugs in history, has become most intensively studied— while readily available treatments are hardly studied at all. . . . Patients want studies of treatments which could be made available to all, not only those with money or insurance.
>
> The Community Research Alliance [like New York's CRI] is committed to having effective PWA representation on all decision-making bodies: the Institutional Review Board (IRB), the Scientific Advisory Committee, and the board of directors.

The planning board appointed Tom Wilcox full-time administrator. He had recently moved to San Francisco from New York, where he had been manager of the PWA Health Group. CRA organized an institutional review board and a scientific advisory committee in preparation for carrying out clinical trials.

By the summer of 1989, having experienced an impetus from the commendation of the Presidential Commission, CRI had gained the participation of 190 New York physicians; nine trials were under way involving more than 500 patients; and CRI annual budget had reached $1 million. In San Francisco, CRA had assembled thirty volunteers on various boards and committees and had initiated a monitoring project with a plant long used in herbal medicine and was exploring possible collaboration with pharmaceutical companies in research projects.

AIDS and the Social Crisis

O n the February 28, 1989 PBS television program "The Education of Admiral Watkins," the Admiral admitted that before his Commission experience he "had no idea of the link between what is now defined as the underclass and AIDS. I didn't realize the suffering, the agony, the rejection, the denial were building, were hardening in the underclass."

A stream of witnesses at April 1988 hearings on societal and legal issues helped to educate Admiral Watkins and the other Commissioners. Dr. Erol Ricketts of the Rockefeller Foundation warned that "the spread of AIDS in the intravenous drug population and its maintenance in that population is predicated on the emergence and growth of the underclass and the drug subculture within the underclass since the 1960s. The growth of the underclass has served as a breeding ground for the spread of AIDS."

Dr. Ronald Mincy summarized an Urban Institute study that characterized underclass neighborhoods as having "a very high incidence of welfare dependent families, female-headed households, males who were out of the labor force for more than three quarters of the year and a very high rate of high school dropouts in the teenage population." Census data, he noted, did not provide a measure of crime and drug abuse, problems endemic in such neighborhoods. The underclass, the study found, "is almost entirely an urban population . . . 60 percent black and 10 percent Hispanic." He pointed out that the 750,000 estimated to be in the underclass in 1970 had grown to two and a half million in 1980.

Various witnesses advised that special problems are' posed in educating the underclass on AIDS issues because of their suspicion of authority figures and the different language and mores among the underclass. Minority researchers and social workers would have to be trained to reach them.

Nathaniel M. Semple, vice president and secretary of the Research and Policy

Committee of the Committee for Economic Development, "a business group whose membership consists of chief executive officers and top business leaders and academics from around the country" (including Admiral Watkins), advised the Commission that "forty percent of the net new increase in the labor force between 1985 and the year 2000 [would] be from the minority community, a substantial fraction of whom [would] have grown up with special needs and in poverty." He spoke of "the real fear [that] our nation is developing a truly permanent underclass, individuals who lack all the tools to become full participants in society." The committee had determined that efforts "must begin with pregnancy and health counseling of teenagers . . . and it involves the needs of education and especially the risk of AIDS. . . . these children of children who are also having children now face the reality of the threat of an epidemic they do not understand."

The cost of programs to deal with this crisis the committee set as "at least $11 billion a year and . . . even higher."

The critical social problems providing the environment for the spread of the AIDS epidemic that were exposed during the Presidential Commission hearings affected far broader segments of the population than the underclass.

Unemployment

The Reagan administration boasted of the creation of 17 million new jobs during its eight years in office and of a reduction in the rate of unemployment to less than 6 percent (approximately 7 million adults). On September 27, 1987 the *New York Times* offered, however, an alternate view, estimating that between 10 and 20 million Americans in their prime working years formed a hard core of nonworkers. These people, the *Times* pointed out, were not counted as unemployed by the Labor Department because they were not actively seeking jobs.

Dr. Harvey Brenner, a participant in a Johns Hopkins University study undertaken for the Joint Economic Commission of Congress, advised the Commission that "unemployment, declines in income and high school dropout rates are significant predictors of narcotics arrest rates. . . . improvements in health, mental health and longevity and criminal justice indices are related to per capita income and decreased rates." Brenner believed that "the extraordinary social costs associated with the poverty population, including heroin abuse and related AIDS," required the identification of "general policy options, among these, investment in education, retraining of the unstably employed and unemployed and a national commitment to a full and meaningful employment policy." This problem, he continued, "is related to much of the AIDS problem."

(Dr. Brenner's full-employment proposal evoked no comment from members of the Commission and was not incorporated in the Commission's Final Report.)

Michael Frye, president of the board of STRIVE, an East Harlem employment service, noted that he was testifying precisely on the day on which twenty years earlier riots had broken out nationally following upon the assassination of Martin Luther King. "Maybe AIDS," he suggested, "is the riots of the '80s to force us again to deal with an issue that we have not dealt with, that is, finding ways to help people become employed, become independent, get off welfare and feel some kind of self-worth."

Responding to these pessimistic prognostications, Admiral Watkins recalled that upon the replacement of the draft by voluntary recruitment the Navy succeeded in bringing 70 percent of the youth at risk into the mainstream through an integrated and comprehensive rehabilitation program that included health education and health promotion along with motivational regimes to provide career orientation and the building of self-esteem.

Almost a year later, however, on the PBS program Watkins admitted: "I just wasn't exposed to this other side of life. I've been in the closed womb of the military. I learned a great deal about society and softened some of my military views in working on the other side of society's aisle. The military was a lot easier."

Homelessness

According to a January 22, 1988 NBC television documentary, of a total number of homeless estimated as high as 3 million, 300,000 were children wandering homeless on the streets and another 250,000 were Viet Nam veterans. A September 1988 estimate, however, by the national Network of Runaway and Youth Services in Washington put the number at approximately 1.2 million runaway and "throwaway" children. Supporting themselves by prostitution, a large percentage of the homeless children represented a dangerous source for expansion of the AIDS epidemic.

In January 1988 Dr. Ernest Drucker of the Montefiore Hospital reported to the Commission that 10 percent of the AIDS patients in the Bronx were homeless. Many, he declared, were "afraid to go to hospitals because once they are diagnosed as having AIDS, they cannot be discharged to shelters."

In September of that year ten of thirteen experts on a National Academy of Sciences commission established to study the needs of the homeless felt so frustrated at the Academy's insistence upon a bland and "objective" style in the official report that they published a supplement to the report in which they voiced their "sense of shame and anger" at the plight of the homeless. "Contemporary American homelessness," the statement declared, "is an outrage, a national scandal" that required expression in more than "a careful, sophisticated and dispassionate analysis . . . its tragedy demands something more direct and human, less qualified and detached . . . anger and dismay." The statement expressed uneasiness because "of our inability to state the most basic recommendation: Homelessness in the United States is an inexcusable disgrace and must be eliminated."

Illiteracy and Youth Problems

On July 27, 1988 a study published by the National Geographic Society and widely publicized in the media reported that of eight industrialized nations investigated for knowledge of geography and current events, the United States ranked third from last among adults but decisively last among 18- to-24-year-olds. Seventy-five percent of Americans could not locate the Persian Gulf and two-thirds could not find Viet Nam on a map; almost half the population were unaware of a conflict between Arabs and Israelis and a similar number could not identify the country in which there was a conflict between Sandinistas and Contras; 45 percent could not identify South Africa as the country practicing apartheid; half could not locate the state of Illinois on a map or approximate the population of the United States; and 5 percent did not know that Washington was the capital of the nation.

A National Assessment of Educational Progress found that of the 2.4 million who graduate annually from high schools, "as many as 25 percent cannot read and write at the eighth-grade or 'functionally literate' level." The report made no mention of the additional 25 percent who drop out before graduation.

Andrea R. Bowden, supervisor of science and health education for the Baltimore school system, expressed concern about providing AIDS education to school dropouts "at high risk in becoming involved in drug abuse and other dangerous behaviors." She noted that "young people are being bombarded with confusing messages. While society and the media seem to condone irresponsible sex and drug use, children are advised to 'say no.'"

Of sexual promiscuity, with its attendant dangers in the spread of AIDS, Congressman Ted Weiss declared to the Commission: "We have had statistics that by the age of 17 some 50 percent of teenagers have been sexually active and by the age of 19 the numbers are in excess of 70 and 75 percent. The field is there for the spread of the disease unless our young people are impressed with the knowledge as to why they really have to behave themselves in a responsible way."

Nathaniel M. Semple, representing the Committee for Economic Development, called attention to the fact that "nearly one-third of sexually active teenagers use no contraception whatsoever . . . and virtually no teenage boys practice contraception, and to the extent that AIDS is transmitted heterosexually, this exposes these teenagers to the risk of AIDS."

Providing a warning as to the possible spread of AIDS among teenagers and young adults is the rapid rise in sexually transmitted diseases. According to an Institute of Medicine report, "For 1987, a 30 percent increase in syphilis was reported in the United States, primarily among heterosexuals. . . . In addition, the areas reporting the largest absolute increase in syphilis cases (i.e., Florida, New York City and California) were also areas that have high rates of HIV infection."

As of the spring of 1988, according to CDC statistics (certainly incomplete), AIDS cases among adolescents represented a mere 1 percent of the total, but the number of cases was doubling each year. The 20–29-year age group, however, represented more than 20 percent of those infected with the virus, many of whom had been infected during adolescence.

In a report entitled "AIDS and the Adolescent" prepared for the Commission, Karen Hein, director of the Adolescent AIDS Program at the Albert Einstein College of Medicine, noted that the sex ratio among adolescent AIDS patients was 2.1 males to 1 female as against the national average of 15 to 1, with minority groups representing 58 percent of the cases. Among the 503 cases of AIDS officially reported among adolescents as of January 1988, "the total number of cases was lower for homosexual/ bisexual (44 percent) and higher for the IVD category (23 percent)" than the national average.

It is among the youth—ill-educated and inadequately prepared for productive participation in the national economy, deprived of a common cultural heritage and ignorant of the history and best traditions of this country and of heroes worthy of emulation—it is this intellectually deprived and morally disarmed generation that confronts the threat of AIDS most immediately. With little sense of self-worth and few prospects for an adult life that offers satisfactions beyond the pursuit of greed and personal power, millions of young people have turned to drugs, alcohol, promiscuous sexuality and wanton violence.

The association of poverty, the drug culture and the school dropout rate was graphically represented to the Commission by Dr. Ricketts of the Rockefeller Foundation:

> How do you tell kids in poor neighborhoods to stay in school and get an
> education with the alternative mode of mobility that they see around them. They
> see people spend three years in the drug economy, and they are driving fancy
> cars and they have lots of money, and with a high school education it is next to
> impossible to acquire those things in a lifetime. So we have what is being
> promoted by the drug economy as an alternative mode of achievement in the
> United States, and that is perhaps one of the most corrosive aspects in terms of
> the drug subculture and economy, posing an alternative mode of achievement in
> the country.

Crime and Violence

Alone among the industrialized nations, the United States accepts violence as a natural phenomenon of daily life, and 48 percent of the nation's households own a firearm. "Homicides in some of the nation's largest cities," reported the *New York Times* on January 15, 1987, "rose sharply in 1986 as officials grappled with an increase in shootings among teenagers and a seemingly intractable spread of cocaine and its derivative, crack." Of 10,289,609 individuals arrested for crimes in 1986, 585,745 were under 15 years of age; 1,762,539, under 18; and 3,230,653 under 21.

A 1985 FBI record of 87,340 rapes (approximately 239 per day), for example, did not include victims below 16 years of age and included only cases reported to the police. A national study of college women in 1986–1987 disclosed that the number of cases of rape appeared to be ten to fifteen times more common than official government figures stated.

AIDS, Minorities and Drug Abuse

All of these social problems—unemployment, hunger, homelessness and a pervasive atmosphere of sexual promiscuity, crime and violence—provide the environment in which AIDS develops and spreads. But the worst of the social ills and the most important factor in the current spread of AIDS is drug addiction, an evil against which the nation has been waging a losing battle.

In September 1985 President and Mrs. Reagan solemnly proclaimed that "the cancer of drug abuse menaces American society," and Mrs. Reagan urged young people to "just say no." A month later, Reagan signed a comprehensive $1.7 billion antidrug bill for "a national crusade against drugs, a sustained relentless effort to rid America of this scourge."

Associating the president's proclamation of a "national crusade" against drugs with the AIDS crisis, the Institute of Medicine (IOM) in its 1986 report, "Confronting AIDS," called for an "expansion of the system for treating IV drug use. Thorough treatment," the document declared, "for users who have not been infected with HIV could greatly reduce their chances of being infected, and users who have already been infected would be less likely to infect others." IOM noted that "at a purely economic level, treating AIDS costs from $50,000 to $150,000 per case, whereas drug abuse treatment costs as little as $3,000 per patient per year in non-residential programs."

The president's national crusade, like "new" AIDS therapy programs inaugurated with fanfare by FDA and NIH, proved to be more a public relations venture than an actuality. In February 1987 Senator Alfonse D'Amato of New York and other Congressional critics were voicing outrage at the president's proposed cuts of more than $900 million in the 1988 antidrug budget.

At Commission hearings on November 24 Cardinal O'Connor exclaimed: "I get frustrated when I ask myself if we are taking drugs seriously or if we are just throwing up our hands, and there is no answer."

At the mid-December hearings of the Commission Dr. J. Besteman, executive director of the Alcohol and Drug Problems Association, expressed concern that "the drug abuse treatment system [would] . . . by default become a hospice system for addicts with AIDS." He noted that despite the fact that personnel of publicly funded projects are paid "modest salaries to work with the most debilitated and difficult patients, an extraordinary level of caring and energy was being expended by staff and other patients on behalf of the AIDS patients receiving drug treatment. As that number grows," he warned, "and the service demands expand, the drug treatment functions are in danger of being overwhelmed."

Dr. Erol Ricketts warned the Presidential Commission that "if AIDS continues within the IV drug abuser population, it will certainly decimate numerous minority males and hence have a significant impact on the demography of the minority population in the years to come."

In September 1987 the *New York Times* reported estimates ranging from 17 to 37 percent in the rate of AIDS infection among New York State's 43,000 prisoners. A study in October 1987 by the National Institute of Justice reported a cumulative total of 1,964 confirmed AIDS cases in seventy federal, state and local correction systems that responded to the study—a 156 percent increase in the two years since the Institute's first survey.

According to "Transmission of Human Immunodeficiency Virus Infection in the United States," a study by Martha F. Rogers published in the *Report of the Surgeon General's Workshop on Children with HIV Infection and Their Families of April 6–9, 1987,* "Over half (65 percent) of reported cases of AIDS in women, 69 percent of heterosexual men with AIDS and 73 percent of the perinatally acquired AIDS cases in children were related to IV drug abuse or sexual contact with IV drug abusers . . . the majority . . . black or Hispanic . . . most . . . inner-city dwellers of low socioeconomic status."

In an article entitled "Intravenous Drug Abuse and Women's Medical Issues" appearing in the same workshop report, Dr. Constance B. Wofsy pointed out that "78 percent of women with AIDS are between the ages of 13 and 39, the peak childbearing ages. . . . There may be 200,000 women who carry the virus of the 1–2 million Americans infected."

In his keynote address to the April 1987 Workshop on Children with HIV Infection, Surgeon General C. Everett Koop insisted that as many as 12,000 additional children above the 3,000 estimated by CDC "are reported to show symptoms of the infection but do not fit the specific CDC criteria. What we are seeing," Koop concluded,

> . . . is more tragic evidence of high-risk pregnancies and births which are most likely to occur among black women . . . who are poor . . . who are not ready for the world of work . . . who may not even have a high school diploma . . . and who do not have ready access to good prenatal and perinatal health care. This additional catastrophic news for the black community, already under great economic and social stress . . . is . . . more evidence of the apparent inability of American society in general to make much headway in helping these young women deal with their own sexuality and their own destinies.

Barbara Blum, president of New York City's Foundation for Child Development, sketched for the Commission the complex problems of dealing with pediatric AIDS cases. Among the additional personnel required, she said, to care for pediatric AIDS cases besides home health aides, homemakers and practical and registered nurses is a case manager with a caseload of no more than ten babies at a time, "responsible for coordinating all necessary services for boarder babies and their families and for acting as a liaison with the child welfare system to secure placement for the child."

For a group home, less costly than other facilities, "besides a director there must be teachers, teacher assistants, bus escorts, a full-time nurse and social worker, a part-time medical director and some auxiliary help from a hospital. Furthermore, society must either provide a wide range of support services to assure the emotional, economic and practical capacity of natural parents, relatives or foster parents for the care of the infants."

◆ ◆ ◆

Interviewed on March 23, 1988 Commissioner Dr. Burton Lee declared, "The more I see, the more I've heard in the hearings, the more it has been impressed upon me that drug abuse is the main health problem that we have in the United States today." To Colleen Conway-Welch, the testimony in the hearings revealed that "the bleakness was greater than I expected with the children in IV drug abuse." In the Final Report of the Commission, a sizable percentage of the recommendations would be devoted to the drug addiction aspect of the AIDS crisis.

Homophobia and Discrimination

A Gallup Poll in July 1987 revealed that 42 percent of respondents, including 57 percent of Evangelicals, agreed that persons with AIDS were suffering "a divine punishment" and that they had "only themselves to blame." Two months later, responding to these right-wing elements, Senator Lowell Weicker declared to the Commission: "Everyone wants to know how much money we are spending on AIDS in America. Has anyone ever asked how much we are spending on syphilis or gonorrhea or any other venereal disease that is associated with the "straight practices?" . . . I would have been just as insulted over that question as I am over this question."

A major argument of homophobic right-wingers against appropriation of special funds to combat HIV infection is that the disease affects far fewer people than cancer or heart disease. In its 1988 Update of "Confronting AIDS," the Institute of Medicine rebutted such assertions with a series of arguments:

> No one disease, past or present, encompasses all the challenges posed by AIDS.
> AIDS is an infectious, fatal disease for which there is now no cure. All infected persons appear to remain infectious, both during the long asymptomatic incubation period of HIV infection and during symptomatic disease.
> The primary sufferers of AIDS come from what is ordinarily a healthy and productive population group: young adults. . . . AIDS has moved from 13th in 1984 to 8th leading cause of premature mortality in 1986, according to CDC. The absolute mortality caused by AIDS to date may be exceeded by other major diseases, but the steep slope of its rise and the youth of its victims are unmatched.
> These social constructions of disease, and the fertile ground they provide

for restrictive or discriminatory social responses, also set AIDS apart as a matter of special concern.

Attempts to control the disease by traditional public health measures are complicated by the fact that AIDS first occurred in already stigmatized groups—homosexual men and intravenous (IV) drug abusers—and the social response to the disease has been confounded by moralistic assignments of blame. A further compelling reason to direct special attention toward AIDS is that it is preventable by modifying the behavior that brings people into contact with the virus.

AIDS has not only brought fear and grief to the gay community but also posed a genuine tragedy "in the history of the male homosexual," Dr. Brenner of Johns Hopkins University observed to the Commission. "The AIDS epidemic," he noted, followed upon a period of greater tolerance and "brought not only a horrific form of death but a return of much of the social taboo and stigma against self-identification of homosexuals."

Indeed, since the spread of the AIDS epidemic, gays and lesbians have increasingly been victims of violence. In June 1988, following upon several especially vicious local incidents, David Wertheimer, executive director of the New York City Gay and Lesbian Anti-Violence Committee, announced that the number of cases of homophobic assaults during the first six months of 1988 was 35 percent higher than during the same period a year earlier. Of the 309 reported incidents, "13 were murders, 61 were assaults by strangers and 55 were attacks that took place in homosexuals' homes, often by family members. . . . Last year," said Wertheimer, "we were more likely to see people struck or punched. This year, we're getting more and more cases of physical assault with a real weapon, like a knife, a gun or a bat."

Regarding a poll taken in Pennsylvania with similar results, the Task Force of the Philadelphia Gay and Lesbian Anti-Violence Committee commented: "The absence of civil rights protection at the state and federal level exacerbates the growing problem of anti-gay and anti-lesbian violence. The fear of revictimization by authorities and the implicit threat of public disclosure discourages gay and lesbian people from reporting incidents of violent victimization."

"Fears of the societal response" because of the "public hysteria and social stigma attached to AIDS," Dr. William M. Mitchell of Vanderbilt University told the Commission, have resulted in "reluctance . . . to undergo AIDS anti-body testing and a frontal assault on the concept of routine testing."

Homophobia and the Presidential Commission

In his opening remarks at February hearings of the Commission, Admiral Watkins declared:

Last November two persons with AIDS appeared before our Commission in Florida to talk about the need for further research in drug development.

Unfortunately, those two persons with AIDS James Sammone and Patrick Haney have since died of AIDS. I have talked with the fathers of these two young men, and they, in turn, have dedicated their lives to furthering AIDS research on behalf of their sons. So it is in behalf of persons like James Sammone and Patrick Haney and their families that we begin our work today.

One of the principal initial objections of the AIDS community to the Presidential Commission was that various appointees to the Commission had publicly expressed antipathy to homosexuals. "You would think these people might be intolerant," admitted Frank Hagan, media consultant for the Commission, of the conservative commissioners. He had found, however, that "to them homosexuality was just another way of living. It's a shame that the rest of the world couldn't be like the Commission office."

Learning that Commissioner Burton Lee wanted to meet with members of the gay community, Hagan assembled some thirty-five people at his home. Lee subsequently recommended him for a position on the Commission staff, and Hagan helped organize site visits to gay organizations and to assemble AIDS community witnesses for the various Commission hearings.

"As the only gay person on the Commission," said Frank Lilly, not so glowing in his reactions to some of his colleagues as Hagan,

> I have asked questions that would not otherwise have been asked. I think, however, that my main contribution is simply being there. I have a feeling that the homophobia inherent in conservatism, and certainly many of the commissioners are conservative, would have made it easier to run roughshod over many issues. My presence has made that more difficult, though not impossible. [Homophobia] is another crisis area that overlaps with AIDS. Maybe half the members of the Commission recognize that fact. The other half don't want to give up their right to discriminate against homosexuals. On the other hand, a large number of people who have testified before the Commission have spontaneously or under my prodding made the point that homophobia is a factor in AIDS.

Dean Conway-Welch, who had suffered the loss of a close friend through AIDS, was surprised to discover "how people have taken this disease and embedded it in their value systems. People who express very certain views about homosexuality," she said, "see AIDS as another underpinning for their fears. People with a more humanistic commitment to social issues feel about AIDS the way they feel about polio or tuberculosis or the common cold."

On the wall of her office, Peggy Dufour, a senior staffer, posted photographs of many of the PWA witnesses. "They made a tremendous impact," she said. "They made you see it can happen to anyone, any time, anywhere. How do you struggle against it, how do you maintain your dignity, how do you believe every day that you have to go on. Working with Philip [the gay office worker]," she said, "has been a great inspiration for all of us, too."

"I will not forget Clarence Kane [a witness before the Commission]," said

Dufour. "First he lost his job in a law firm because of discrimination. Then he lost his town house in Washington and was living on the street. You listen to this and you get filled with absolute rage. No matter how his court case is resolved, it's going to be resolved long after he's dead. All the benefits that we're all working for and will achieve through this report will not be soon enough for so many people."

Admiral Watkins admitted that as Commission chairman he had had his first long conversation with a gay man with AIDS. The large majority of the gay witnesses as well as those he encountered during on-site visits impressed him as thoughtful, serious and able to separate issues regarding the virus from issues regarding homosexual life style. "Their knowledge of the immune system and what was going on in their bodies," he declared, "was greater than that of the average doctor."

When Frank Lilly asked for hearings on homophobia and gay rights, however, "I told him," reported the Admiral, "that I thought such a hearing would be devastating to a report that otherwise was certain to have a powerful impact. It was my opinion, as I stated early on to all the Commission members, including Frank, that if this Commission wandered into that no man's land, did something that the president's mandate did not permit, we would emasculate what should be in this report, which is so powerful as to what this nation has to do." The Admiral added that for such an investigation he would have to involve Cardinal O'Connor and the Dannemeyers. (Frank Dannemeyer, a California congressman, had sponsored legislation blatantly discriminatory against people with HIV infection.) The topic invited discussion also of issues that the Commission frankly was not qualified to deal with.

"Time and time again," the Admiral recounted,

> we chatted with the gay leaders about the degree to which we should involve ourselves in the issue of gay rights. It was clear to the executive director of GMHC, the leadership in the National Coalition on AIDS and many others that we would serve all in the nation far better by keeping those issues separate and go after the virus, solve that problem, deal with discrimination issues in connection with the virus, concerning ourselves with those that were infected, deal with the confidentiality issues, with housing, with job loss.

At an executive session on June 6, when the Commission was winding down its operation, the Admiral related:

> Dr. Crenshaw [a Commissioner who at the time of her appointment had been attacked as a particularly vicious homophobe] raised her hand and said, "I think we should have hearings on homophobia." Lilly, who was sitting next to Dr. Crenshaw, took the microphone. He said that while he would like to have such a session he felt it was inappropriate in the context of the Commission's work. Frank would never have reached that conclusion without the thorough discussions we had had on discrimination, on confidentiality in records, on the litigious atmosphere, on the sloppiness in drug development. I called Frank and congratulated him on his courage in disagreeing with Dr. Crenshaw. He said, "It was hard for me to do it."
>
> Discrimination and follow-up actions by the president on discrimination

were the only two areas on which I felt we were going to have deep, substantive disagreements within the Commission.

The Admiral considered the Cardinal's vote, in particular, in doubt. "Obviously, the Cardinal Archbishop of New York," said the Admiral, "devoted to the Holy Father, is going to be rigid on certain things. Where was this Commission going to take him in ideology and morality?" Cardinal O'Connor gave the Admiral his proxy and empowered him to vote affirmatively on the issue.

The Admiral considered it critical that John Creedon (president and chief executive officer of the Metropolitan Life Insurance Company and one of the most conservative of the commissioners) vote with the yes voters. He did so.[1]

"Even though opposed to the Commission's stance," the Admiral noted, "Penny Pullen [another of those considered most prejudiced against gays] helped draft the discrimination section of the Final Report. . . . She wrote no minority report in opposition though she was capable of composing a minority report that could have been damaging."

The night before the final vote, the Admiral said to Pullen privately:

Penny, I believe we are going to vote for an affirmative position on anti-discrimination. . . . Are you going to be politically embarrassed? Is there anything I can do to mitigate that? She replied, "I'm not going to be embarrassed." When a reporter asked her whether she had voted against the proposition, she replied, "I didn't vote." To my way of thinking that was a sign of movement.

If at the beginning, on October 7, we had asked each commissioner to write down his opinion on the issue, we would not have had the vote in favor of confidentiality, the 8 out of 13 vote on anti-discrimination, the discussion of partner notification. . . . Almost every one of our recommendations represents a growth recommendation [from] nine months of listening to six hundred people. The evidence was so compelling as to what beset the nation.

Over the nine months, all the Commissioners, including me, grew immensely, to the extent where we were willing to back off from ideological nicks we had to start with.

---

[1] The Admiral may not have realized, indeed, how far Creedon had moved as a result of his experiences on the Commission. On September 14, 1988 Creedon delivered a commentary on the first of a series of Metropolitan Life Insurance Company AIDS documentaries on ABC network television. He declared:

We have learned . . . that [AIDS] is a disease that if left unchecked could threaten the well-being of our entire society. . . . we know how it is transmitted and how the virus attacks the body. With this knowledge we can take proper steps to protect ourselves and those we love. . . . And with knowledge we can better understand the tragedies the AIDS virus generates for people in different walks of life. . . . All of us need to commit our energies in defeating AIDS. If we can put aside our philosophical differences and accept the challenges of AIDS, it could be one of our finest hours as a caring people.

CHAPTER

The Report of the Presidential Commission

In interviews held when the Presidential Commission was either approaching the end of its assignment or actually winding up its affairs, five Commissioners (including the Commission chairman) and several members of the staff were asked to respond to the following proposition: "In light of the numerous critical and seemingly intractable problems confronting our society—homelessness, hunger, illiteracy, unemployment, violence, drug abuse and a crisis in health services—a resolution of the AIDS crisis seems unlikely."

Before being confronted with this proposition, Dr. Burton Lee III had spoken about "the problems we have in dealing with the people in our society who need the help the most. In particular," he said, "I'm talking about the children, about the children on the streets, the children who are prostitutes and drug addicts, drug abusers in their early teens, a group that has really caught my sympathies tremendously. We're simply not addressing the problems in this country in any kind of meaningful way." Posed with the proposition, however, Lee responded with a more partisan viewpoint. He objected to any characterization of the Reagan administration as "dilatory and lethargic" in its response to the AIDS crisis and criticized instead "the fighting in [the Democrat-controlled] Congress about budgetary requirements, about gay rights and about how much to commit to drug abuse."

Violence Lee attributed to the widespread possession of arms. "You have an enormous number of people in the United States who don't agree with us," he declared. "The gun lobby is incredible."

Regarding homelessness, which he characterized as a "relatively new problem that has come upon the American consciousness," Lee was hopeful. It was a problem "currently being addressed." Democracies, he asserted, react to problems rather than dealing with them prospectively. Unemployment he said required "a twenty-two hour discussion. You have a tremendous number of women in the work force, some of whom don't want to work full time. . . . You have to break unemployment down to talk about it." Admitting that the number of unemployed was too great, he was of the opinion that some unemployment was inevitable "unless you're going to be China or Russia and run an absolutely socialist economy in which everybody will get something to do, no matter whether it's just pushing a rock from one side of the road to the other, and you pay a penalty for that kind of society."

On the other hand, according to Lee,

> in the inner city areas, the husband almost doesn't exist. . . . If you give these men jobs so that we don't have forty percent unemployed in these segments of the male population, or even higher, the women will start marrying them again. . . . They will stop being welfare dependents. . . . And that is going to be one of our recommendations, if I can possibly do it, in our final report. . . . You have to rebuild the infrastructure of America. If you have to put in a WPA to provide jobs, so be it!

Asked whether such a proposal did not represent the Russian–Chinese way, Lee replied: "Well, there is a hard core of people in any country that you have to deal with."

What could the Presidential Commission hope to accomplish?

> I expect to be able to do something because this is a Presidential Commission. . . . I am not saying that I am an optimist. I am saying that I still want to give it a shot. In a dilemma like we're in, you'll find, in general, people rising to do their best. We have certain people on our Commission that have done that, and we are running the show, and this Commission is going to come out with good material. . . . We're going to finish our report as fast as we can and hope that somebody else is going to pick up the ball. I think [this report] is going to end up being different from what people expected—bipartisan, sympathetic and substantive.

Confronted with the proposition as to whether a resolution of the AIDS crisis was possible within the general crises in American society, Dean Colleen Conway-Welch replied, "I guess it depends upon your definition of resolution. It's a very bleak picture that you paint of our current society. I think there is another side to it. Part of the resolution is that we are learning about many of those bleak variables and learning about them because of AIDS. If anything, I think that AIDS has served a useful purpose at least in focusing us on these ills in a way that has not happened before." On the other hand, according to Welch, it had been a constant concern of Commission members that they were fluctuating between focusing on AIDS and focusing on the whole society. To be meaningful, the final report had both to be germane to AIDS, she said, and to deal with the infrastructure of problems in creating an environment that must be dealt with in conjunction with dealing with AIDS.

Posed with the proposition, Frank Lilly responded:

That's a loaded question. Certainly we have not done well with the drug
problem. The Commission has come up with some recommendations. . . . I
don't think AIDS is going to go away unless we come up with an effective and
cheap vaccine, and that's not likely in my lifetime. If we come up with one, it's
likely to be too expensive to ship around to millions of people in Africa. In
public lectures I have said that we are not going to solve the AIDS problem until
we solve the drug problem and vice versa. I have said the same thing about
homophobia because that's another area that overlaps eventually with AIDS.

Like the Commissioners interviewed, Tom Brandt, the Commission's press officer, responded with measured optimism to the proposition. "We have to do the best
we can," he declared.

What we can accomplish is another issue. As we have gotten into the study of
the AIDS epidemic, we have turned up this rock, then that. We have found it's
all interlinked and co-factored with all the other issues. The drug issue is
probably going to be the area of our main emphasis. The health delivery system
at some point in four years, eight years, may reach a crisis. Terrible problems
are emerging—financial problems, people being missed, people being
bankrupted. AIDS is going to stress out an already stressed system.

The Commission, he declared, was charged with the AIDS problem:

We're not charged with all the problems of the world. How far afield do you go
to solve the drug problem before you can solve the AIDS problem? Do you solve
the problem of illiteracy first or poverty first? All you can do is to attempt to
awaken the nation. If you can do that within the full context so that a new level
of discussion is posed, that will be a contribution.

"A researcher who testified before us some months ago," Brandt recalled, "said
something that Admiral Watkins repeats often: 'When I started this, I was a conservative, but when you get into this issue you find that lines between liberal and
conservative disappear.' That," said Brandt, "is what's happening in the Commission."
In regard to the AIDS crisis and its ramifications, Brandt, a conservative Republican,
had become nonpartisan.

Frank Hagan, the Commission's media consultant, openly gay, said that he had
experienced culture shock upon finding out how things were done in government.
For all the difficulties, he was convinced that one person can make a difference. His
first impression of the Commission was that some members were hard-line Repub-
licans. A Republican himself, Hagan says he could "share the viewpoints of people
looking in and looking out." Having had an opportunity to speak with all the members directly, he considered that the Commission breakdown, from the point of view
of the gay community, was 75 percent in the right direction. Unlike others connected
with the Commission, however, Hagan agreed without hesitation that a resolution
of the AIDS crisis was far off, if possible at all, in the context of the general crisis in
the national society.

Alone among the Commissioners and staff members interviewed, Peggy Dufour was unqualifiedly optimistic. "I know," she said, "that in history things do get resolved one way or another. I think we're smarter than to let our civilization fall apart, than to let 30 percent of our people go to waste. I really think that America is waking up to that. Who talked about the underclass even five years ago?" Nevertheless, Dufour posed a fundamental proviso to her optimistic prediction:

> Unless we change the structure of our society, the problems are not going to change. We had a lot of trouble getting our Commission members to agree to discuss social issues. After those hearings were through, they really agreed precisely because of what you're saying. Yes, you can solve this problem, but there's another bigger one and they're all tied together, and how are you going to fix it? It seems to me that people all around the country really want to participate in making their society better.

Reminded that the Commission chairman did not share her confidence, Dufour admitted:

> The Admiral sees it from a political point of view much better than I can. He's been around this city for a long time. He knows the resistance. I see it from the point of view of the people not in this city, people out there who care, people like the volunteers in literacy programs.
> We had encountered so much negativity in New York. . . . I met so many people around the country that are so far behind in the process and are just awakening to the need and to the sensitivities [regarding AIDS]. They're not going to have to go through what New York has gone through. That in itself is really a positive thing. It shows that we don't have to start at zero.

Interviewed on July 20, 1988, after the publication of the Commission's Final Report, Admiral Watkins responded to the proposition without equivocation:

> This is an American problem, not just a question of NIH–FDA. It runs through American society, and if you read our recommendations and read our obstacles to progress, what you're seeing is a society that . . . can no longer be responsive to fast events like the unknowns in HIV. Justice can't respond. HHS can't be in sync with Education, can't work with Defense. . . . The Hill with 60 bills couldn't move any one of them. The state legislatures are all taking different actions. If you look at this entire situation, you see that society is ready for a major structural change in attitudes—serving others instead of self. . . . I really believe this virus has pushed that home to me more than I have ever had it pushed home before.

The Report

In the 1988 Update of its comprehensive 1986 document, "Confronting AIDS," published three weeks before the Commission's Final Report, IOM noted that "the [presidential] commission has made major contributions to the public's understanding of

HIV infection and AIDS and to the development of a compassionate and informed response to the epidemic. Guided by Admiral James D. Watkins's strong leadership and open-minded approach," the IOM document went on to state, "the commission's focused attention has been effective in bringing diverse public and private resources to bear on a national problem."

◆ ◆ ◆

The Commission's Final Report comprised 158 pages divided into twelve chapters, each dealing with a specific aspect of a national strategy against the disease: Incidence and Prevalence; Patient Care; Health Care Providers; Basic Research, Vaccine, and Drug Development; The Public Health System; Prevention; Education; Societal Issues; Legal and Ethical Issues; Financing Health Care; The International Response; Guidance for the Future.

In a "Letter of Transmissal," Admiral Watkins advised the president that Commission members had had

> an unusual opportunity to view contemporary American society through the
> lens of the HIV. . . . the frightening specter of drug abuse and its relation to the
> spread of the virus; an overly burdened and unnecessarily costly health care
> system; a drug development system unresponsive to the fast-changing
> unknowns surrounding this epidemic; absence of integrated health education
> and health promotion programs in our schools; an increasingly litigious and
> adversarial relationship between providers and consumers of health care; and a
> society in which members were still too quick to reject, deny, condemn, and
> discriminate.

As in the Commission's preliminary report and in his previous public statements, Admiral Watkins emphasized the necessity for making "prevention and treatment of intravenous drug abuse . . . a top national priority . . . with greatly expanded treatment capacity, with the goal of treatment on demand, to restore addicted individuals to healthful living." The Admiral noted that the epidemic offered "an opportunity to confront and begin to solve many of the problems our society faces. . . . to turn the goodness that is out there . . . into an unbeatable army against this viral enemy that has captured the early ground."

Representative of what Admiral Watkins called the "goodness . . . out there" in the nation, a vanguard force in the war against the viral enemy, was the Issues Committee of New York ACT UP. Bill Bahlman, the committee's liaison with the Commission, obtained a draft of the Final Report and with the committee went over the document line by line and page by page, noting specific suggestions for transmission to the Commission's staff. Dr. Iris Long of the Issues Committee actually wrote the section on pediatric AIDS that appeared in the Final Report.

Although most of the nearly 600 recommendations in the Report are expressed in bold but precise terms, many are phrased as exhortations, almost as though the commissioners feared to press too hard for fundamental changes necessary for a successful combating of the epidemic. Admiral Watkins explained that the "shoulds," which repeatedly appear in the text, were originally "must," but he said, "I can't use 'must' because that presupposes failure if action is not taken. If you 'should' do it and you don't do it, at least you've only violated the 'should.' The 'must' says you failed if you didn't do it. I said that sometimes you can use 'must,' but not very often."

What emerges implicitly from the Report is a comprehensive exposé of seven years of lack of leadership, of fumbling and indifference. The Report charged that in the HIV crisis the White House through the Office of Management and Budget (OMB) balked congressional will. (Even as White House agencies secretly conducted operations in defiance of the will of the Congress in foreign affairs.) The Report condemned "the inflexibility of OMB regulation of internal resource allocation and program development" and urged that "henceforth OMB . . . not undermine congressional intent."

The Commission was also critical of the Congress. "Several pieces of comprehensive HIV legislation have been introduced and considered," the Report declared, "but none has yet been endorsed by both houses."

Again and again the Report noted insufficiency in funding, even cuts in funding, for agencies suffering a critical shortage of facilities and without "adequate staff at any level to respond to this crisis." The Health Care Financing Administration, for example, had reduced through attrition the number of its laboratory inspectors in the blood industry by 30 percent.

The Report called attention to "the need to free federally sponsored research from bureaucratic restrictions that delay progress and constrain exploration . . . to create new ways of thinking about basic biomedical research and science education . . . to upgrade many of America's aging research facilities and properly equip them for HIV research." The Report noted a need, too, "for greater communication of research results, both within the research community and to the general public" as well as a need for "increased access by a broader spectrum of the infected population to a greater variety of experimental treatments."

The Report called for "a more rapid response by all elements of government . . . to speed NIH research efforts" as well as greater expedition in the assignment of grants, especially those for longer term investigation. The Report saw a danger for the future in "the lack of basic science education programs in elementary and secondary education" and in the insufficiency of training programs on the college and university level "to supply the necessary number of future researchers."

Criticisms and proposals in the Report in regard to the major federal public health agencies exposed the lamentable disarray in the federal response to the AIDS crisis.

The Centers for Disease Control

The Report accused the Centers for Disease Control (CDC) of failing to exert "strong . . . leadership in the public health community for obtaining and coordinating HIV infection data" and for assembling data and models to improve the predictive value of mathematical modeling. CDC bore responsibility for a lack of demographic data for estimating the size of the various population groups as well as for the insufficient data on infectivity, on delay between infection and infectivity, on the efficiency of HIV transmission and on progression from infection to death.

The Report further criticized CDC for an exclusive concentration on full-blown AIDS rather than on the HIV infection at all stages of its evolution. It pointed to a duplication of effort and lack of communication among the eight offices of the agency; a need for a clear statement of the agency's mission; and a failure to plan long-range programs.

The Food and Drug Administration

The Report recommended additional resources and expanded quarters for FDA so that it might have the facilities to accelerate HIV-related applications. The Report charged that the treatment IND program was not working; that there was no centralized information network on the IND program and no office with responsibility for helping physicians through the FDA maze for utilizing the program.

The NDA [new drug application] process, the Report stated, needed to be speeded up through elimination of bureaucratic impediments. The Report called for rapid approval or rejection of diagnostic products currently before FDA or in the developmental pipeline and for shortening of the time frame of Phase II trials. It recommended the funding of an independent scientific organization to conduct a review of safety regulations and to determine whether the regulations should be relaxed for drugs under treatment IND regulations; and it proposed that FDA "hold a conference on the subject of collaborative research and development in drug and vaccine development."

The National Institutes of Health

According to the Report, "our national system of research programming and funding is not equipped to reorganize rapidly in response to an emergency. . . . Innovative initiatives," the Report declared, were urgently needed that would "both maintain scientific integrity and shorten the time of discovery to trial, and from trial to safe and effective treatment use."

The Report noted that bureaucracy surrounding grant applications required that valuable staff time employed in filling out grant applications meant less time for delivery of prevention services; that too few research grants were made to younger investigators and funding was inadequate for new or "unpopular" ideas; and that women, minorities, children, IVDUs and individuals at early stages of HIV infection were not being included in clinical trials. The Report expressed concern that NIH had not developed a hotline to provide doctors and patients with up-to-date clinical trial information.

Health Care Services and Personnel

According to the Report, "the health care delivery system is structurally and financially unprepared to deal with diverse needs of the disease." The Report called attention to the unavailability in many communities of "the full continuum of health services required." The Report charged that shortages of physicians and dentists in underserved areas with an estimated population of 34 million were aggravated by the elimination of National Health Service Corps scholarships, an administration action that would reduce the number of physicians committed to work in such areas from a peak of 3,200 in 1986 to a mere 100 by 1994. Similarly, the rapidly growing shortage of nurses was aggravated by administration fiscal policies.

The Report warned: "The acuity of disease of persons with HIV infection, the complexity of their physical and psycho-social needs, the high fatality rate, and the fear of exposure to HIV, along with low salaries and understaffing . . . create a potential for considerable stress, burn-out, turnover, and dramatic projected shortages for the delivery of HIV patient care in the near future."

The Commission called for the elimination of red tape in applications for Medicare, Medicaid and other support programs. In a recommendation surprisingly bold from a Commission appointed by the Reagan administration, the Report urged that the secretary of Health and Human Services, "in conjunction with an independent outside body . . . evaluate the problems of financing our overall health care financing and recommend changes to achieve access to and provision of health care for all segments of our society." (This statement almost represented a call for a national health service!)

Community-Based Organizations (CBOs)

The Report gave generous recognition to community-based programs of comprehensive services developed "largely through the intensive efforts of [the] homosexual community." The Report praised the Community Research Initiative of New York for offering "the possibility to combine the technical expertise of the research community with the outreach potential of community health clinics and physicians in community practice . . . and . . . [to] increase the access of [underrepresented] populations to experimental treatment." The Commission urged funding of community-based organizations, training of community physicians and involvement of community groups in the planning and execution of clinical trials.

(While the Final Report was being drafted, Polly Gault, the energetic executive director of the Commission, learned that FDA Commissioner Frank Young had persuaded Senator Orin Hatch to insist upon the omission from an omnibus AIDS bill sponsored by Hatch and Ted Kennedy of a $5 million subsidy for community-based research. Gault called Young and shouted at him for adding his voice in opposition to the subsidy. Admiral Watkins followed with an equally severe telephone call. As a result of their interventions a $6 million subsidy was included in the bill.)

Discrimination

Exemplifying the general tone of humanity in the Report is the following declaration:

> Each act of discrimination . . . diminishes our society's adherence to the
> principles of justice and equality. Our leaders at all levels . . . should speak out
> against ignorance and injustice and make clear to the American people that
> discrimination against persons with HIV infection will not be tolerated.

"As long as discrimination occurs," the Commission warned, "and no strong national policy with rapid and effective remedies against discrimination is established, individuals who are infected with HIV will be reluctant to come forward for testing, counseling, and care."

Noting that there was not "a societal standard or national policy statement clearly and unequivocally stating that discrimination against persons with HIV infection is wrong," the Report called upon the president to "issue an executive order banning discrimination on the basis of handicap, with HIV infection included as a handicapping condition."

Intravenous Drug Abuse

Numerous recommendations in the Final Report exposed the bankruptcy of the National Crusade against Drugs initiated by the president three years earlier. "Our drug problem pervades all elements of society," the Report warned. "Without a coordinated and sustained response, America as a whole faces a bleak future."

The Report called for a national policy of providing "treatment on demand" for IVD abusers, with an expansion of treatment capacity by 20 percent through the addition of 2,500 new facilities and the training of 59,000 persons as drug abuse workers along with research in behavior change among drug abusers.

Societal Issues

In the introduction to the section on social issues, the report declared that as the Commission proceeded in its investigation of patterns of HIV infection, "the relationship between the spread of HIV and longstanding societal problems became apparent. It is imperative that this nation recognize and address the context in which the epidemic is occurring." High indices of HIV infection, the Report noted, are found in neighborhoods—particularly minority neighborhoods—with "high rates of teenage pregnancy, high school dropouts, crime (particularly drug-related crime), welfare dependency, males who are jobless, and female-headed houses." The spread of the epidemic, the Report noted, was occurring disproportionately within the underclass. "Persistent poverty in the midst of an affluent society," it warned, "engenders hopelessness and despair which can lead to heroin abuse and related high rates of crime."

The Report called for "intensive efforts . . . to train and place unskilled workers, including rehabilitated drug addicts, and to build their self-respect, confidence, and hope." On the other hand, according to the Report, "the HIV epidemic provides a unique impetus to address these problems in total rather than continue the piecemeal, fractured, and largely ineffective approach that is being undertaken today." The Report called upon "the nation's business leadership [to] convene a highly visible conference bringing together national corporate and foundation leaders and leaders of regional and community philanthropic organizations."

Learning from Others

In a chapter entitled "The International Response," the Report provided a summary of the state of the AIDS crisis in other nations and offered recommendations for U.S. participation in international research and other activities.

(Regarding the failure to note lessons to be learned from the French approach to the crisis as described by the official heading the French national effort, Admiral Watkins commented that American chauvinism, exemplified in this omission, was resented abroad. "The attitude is," he said, "that we don't need to learn from anybody. . . . this is one thing we thought needed aggressive attention.")

The Report recommended that the Department of Health and Human Services and FDA "develop a mechanism for working with other nations with similar drug development and control programs to accept their data leading to the approval of experimental drugs for HIV disease to be used in clinical trials."

A Permanent Commission on HIV Infection

The Commission proposed the establishment of "some special management oversight entity . . . to see that an action plan to carry out the strategy is aggressively followed . . . to help bring the existing institutional process up to an acceptable level of efficiency in the near term and to remain in being until demonstrated management control over the epidemic is assured." It called upon the president to appoint a seven-member committee to establish "a clear chain of command from the Cabinet to all affected units of the federal government with a single designated official to manage implementation of [the Commission's] Report and related activities within the existing structure." It urged the establishment of a separate Department of Health and "delegation of authority during a declared public health emergency to facilitate procedures which enhance emergency responsiveness including approaches to hiring, acquisition of new space, increases in personnel ceilings, awarding of grants and contracts, regulatory review, and interdepartmental and interagency activities."

According to Bill Bahlman, with perhaps 85 percent of the witnesses expressing similar observations on fundamental social problems associated with AIDS crisis, the Commission was compelled to take the advanced and unequivocal stands expressed in its Final Report. Witnesses sponsored by more conservative members of the Commission, appearing at most of the hearings, quickly discredited themselves by their obvious lack of compassion and of information. Though generally representing no one but themselves, they nevertheless, Bahlman declared, obtained equal play in the press. In Nashville and Indianapolis, outright homophobic testimony made front-page headlines. "Such witnesses," he insisted, "would not have been given any credence at all if the Commission had been composed entirely of top-notch people. The general testimony, however," Bahlman asserted, "was so overwhelming that it would have been outrageous for the Commission to take opposing positions."

Reviewing the Report in the *New York Review of Books* of August 18, 1988, Diane Johnson and Dr. John F. Murray declared:

> One senses in the report a kind of stupefaction, the tone perhaps of an able military administrator seeing for the first time the disorganization and inefficiency of the federal health agencies. . . . Admiral Watkins and his commission understand that drug companies will not develop new drugs without tax incentives and profit; that doctors will not treat with experimental drugs if they are afraid of being sued; that women will not become nurses for low pay and low status; that people without hope of a good life may have little reason to avoid illegal drugs; that people who fear losing jobs and homes will not submit to testing. Therefore, society should address the tax structure, the malpractice laws, the pay and education protection for HIV-infected people, and these are just the beginnings of what would amount to almost a wholesale revision of American society, with its attendant, stupefying costs.

An astute reader would recognize in the Report criticisms and recommendations posed repeatedly by leaders of the AIDS community. Indeed, the congruence of analyses in the Report and those presented by AIDS activists to government agencies, congressional committees and the media and at Commission hearings bespeak the acuity of insight of these dedicated men and women—many infected with the virus or lovers or friends of PWAs—as well as the passionate dedication with which they pressed their demands.

Thus the September–October 1988 Gay Men's Health Crisis newsletter could praise as "progressive" the recommendations in the Report with only a single reservation, regarding criminality of HIV transmission, which, the newsletter claimed, might deter high-risk individuals from seeking testing and counseling.

CHAPTER

The President Receives His Commission's Report

During 1987, with the Irangate disclosures and the increasing uncertainty regarding the national economy, a change began to take place in the national mood. A Gallup Poll in October reported that "the proportion of Americans who believed that victims of AIDS should be treated with compassion [had] jumped to 87 percent, from 78 percent [in July]"; the percentage opposing the right of employers to dismiss people with AIDS rose to 64 percent from 43 percent; and the number opposing quarantining PWAs rose from 51 to 71 percent.

Many in the general population admired the tremendous effort by the gay community to fight for their lives and to care for the afflicted as well as the vigorous pressure mounted by the gay community on all levels of government for action. The assemblage in October of up to half a million gays and lesbians in Washington, unequaled since the days of the civil rights movement, astonished the nation.

The administration, however, ignored the shift in public attitudes. In June 1987 the Justice Department ruled that institutions receiving federal funds could fire or discriminate against PWAs simply because of "fear of contagion" among their employees. In the fall Dr. Otis R. Bowen, secretary of the Department of Health and Human Services, opposed a Congressional bill guaranteeing the civil rights of PWAs. The Social Security Administration began denying disability benefits to PWARCs on the rationale that "they may be dying, but they may not be disabled."

In light of the administration's obduracy, it was understandable that in welcoming Admiral Watkins as a witness at House Subcommittee hearings in April 1988, two months before the publication of the Commission's Final Report, Representative Ted Weiss should express the debt of gratitude owed to him by the nation and the hope Weiss himself harbored—"with not a great deal of optimism"—that even as Watkins had "produced a miracle in managing the Commission he would produce a second miracle" on the basis of the arguments in the documentation assembled by the Commission in persuading the president to implement the Commission's recommendations.

On July 10, two weeks after Admiral Watkins had delivered the Commission's Final Report to the president, at hearings of the Senate Committee on Labor and Human Resources, Senator Edward M. Kennedy also found it necessary to exhort Reagan to respond positively to the recommendations in the Report:

> History will long marvel at the Americans of the 1980s who allowed a virus that cares nothing for our moral preferences to invade our society almost unchecked. . . . It will marvel that we knew our enemy, and it is the virus and not the victims, but wasted precious years and countless lives blaming the sick for their illness. . . . that we already had a workable vaccine, an honest education, but that we allowed children to die while we debated whether or not to tell them the truth. Society can say with near certainty what the virus plans to do for the next ten years. But there is little certainty what our own government plans to do about it.

On July 20, reminded that during the previous six years the president had never taken any action of significance in regard to the epidemic and had rarely even mentioned the AIDS crisis, Admiral Watkins smiled. "The president has thirty days," he remarked. "Then he's supposed to say something about our Report. After the 27th of July," he added enigmatically, "you can make whatever statement you want."

On July 24 Admiral Watkins terminated his duties with the Commission.

On August 1, in response to the Report, the White House issued a ten-point "action plan." Of the ten proposals, two called for further studies, one "emphasize[d the president's] concern" and one was an exhortation to "all sectors of society to respond equitably and compassionately."

"Choosing the weakest of three possible remedies," reported the *New York Times*, "President Reagan today ordered Federal agencies to adopt guidelines that would prevent discrimination in the workplace against employees carrying the AIDS virus." Although calling AIDS "a horrible human problem," the *Times* continued, the president "stopped short of issuing an executive order or endorsing federal anti-discrimination legislation." Instead, he "directed the Attorney General's office to 'conduct an expeditious review' of the Commission's anti-discrimination recommendations."

Commented Henry A. Waxman, chairman of the House Energy and Commerce and Health subcommittee: "First the White House said the Surgeon General would study AIDS. Then the White House said the commission would study AIDS. Now they say the Attorney General will study it. OMB will study it. . . . They hand-pick a commission and . . . don't have the courage to accept its recommendations."

Inasmuch as the Congress over the previous six years had had to force upon the administration larger appropriations than were proposed in presidential budgets, the reaffirmation of the president's "commitment to provide adequate resources . . . to combat the HIV epidemic" seemed less than convincing. His instructions to OMB "to make certain there are no impediments to efficient use of these resources" were directed to an agency that had repeatedly balked Congressional will in regard to AIDS expenditures and policies. The president's order to FDA to "improve labora-tory quality and blood screening tests immediately" would be ineffective without a restoration of the agency's seriously diminished resources.

Perhaps because Admiral Watkins had often emphasized the importance of antidiscrimination legislation and because the president had chosen the weakest option in regard to this problem, the media singled out this issue as though it was the only issue of significance investigated by the Commission. (In fact, the Final Report devoted only 9 of its 158 pages and 35 of its 597 recommendations to this question.)

On the other hand, the president and the media ignored other critical issues that the Admiral singled out in a statement before the July 10 Kennedy Senate committee hearings:

> An over-burdened and overly expensive health care delivery system; a
> terminally slow therapeutic drug development process; an ineffective addressing
> of drug abuse as a significant national threat by all levels of society; the absence
> of an integrated health education and health promotion curriculum in our
> schools and workplaces; a health care professional education process also
> unresponsive to a new, fast moving, and deceptive medical threat; a health care
> delivery system increasingly weakened in quality by shortages of those who
> make the system work; an increasingly litigious and adversarial relationship
> between providers of health care and consumer. . . .

The president totally and the media generally ignored the fifty recommenda-tions in the Report regarding the necessity for confronting the fundamental societal issues providing the environment for the AIDS crisis.

◆ ◆ ◆

In his introduction to ABC's "Nightline" program on the evening of the publication of the president's response to the Final Report, moderator Sam Donaldson declared:

> Mr. Reagan ignored the Commission's recommendation that workers in general
> should not be fired just because they have AIDS. Today Mr. Reagan gave that
> protection only to those who work for the Federal Government. Why did the
> president reject his own commission's advice? A member of the White House
> [Dr. Donald Ian MacDonald, the president's drug policy adviser] said that some
> Administration officials believe that it was 'reward for behavior that causes
> AIDS.' Critics charged that the result is disastrously short of what's needed.

When Dr. MacDonald, the drafter of the ten-point presidential plan and a guest on the program that evening, responded that with states and communities coming up with antidiscrimination laws of their own there was no need for federal legislation, a program commentator intervened to note that only eleven states had laws specifically dealing with AIDS-related discrimination. Even in those states persons could face years of litigation to recover damages, during which time many of them would die.

Also appearing on the "Nightline" program, Commission member Kristine Gebbie found "the president's response disappointing. . . . It suggests further study . . . but fails of following through with federal laws." She pointed out that the Commission's recommendation regarding antidiscrimination legislation was for "a law covering all persons with disability [not just persons with AIDS]." Such a law would establish, she said:

> that persons with HIV infection are no different than a person with epilepsy or
> any other diseases who are currently now protected by a broad level of civil
> rights . . . statutes. . . . Over and over again advocates, physicians, patients said
> without protection discrimination the people we most need to reach with
> education, with testing, with services will not come forward, they are too
> frightened. . . . This is an essential message that they are part of our community,
> that they are a valued part of our society . . . that we will treat them equably,
> taking into account only those things that are relevant to the infection and to
> their health.

Questioned about his statement earlier in the day that a federal law would reward a type of behavior that ought not to be rewarded, MacDonald insisted that he had meant IV drug abusers, not all those infected with HIV. He did admit that "there may be some people in the Administration who want to discriminate against people whose sexual practices they consider amoral."

Gebbie resented the ignoring of most of the proposals in the Final Report. "The recommendations that [were] being put on hold or . . . being treated with the least interest," she charged, "[were] the ones that the Commission saw as most central and ones where the Commission hoped for very strong aggressive presidential response. . . . state governments," she insisted, "will now be given the opportunity to say, well, if the feds are going to study how long it takes to increase [drug] treatment centers, we don't need to rush to find our matching funds to build it up as well."

Regarding the president's disregard of the Commission's recommendation for the appointment of a continuing oversight commission, Gebbie observed that "the chain of command from the president through the cabinet down to every program in the federal government . . . needed to be made much more clear. . . . agencies tripping over each other . . . committees talking about the issues but nobody clearly in charge."

At the conclusion of the program, MacDonald announced with the sanguine confidence characteristic of administration pronouncements about the epidemic:

"The czar in this field today is the president who tends through the directives he sent out today . . . to get these things done."

The tone the following evening in a segment of the PBS "McNeil-Lehrer News Hour" proved quite different from that on "Nightline." Moderator Judy Woodruff began by noting that the president had rejected many of the Commission's nearly 600 recommendations, including the proposal for a new federal antidiscrimination law. He had taken no action on the Commission's recommendation for the appointment of "an AIDS czar"[1] and "did not ask for new funds for treatment for intravenous drug users, the fastest growing group of AIDS victims."

MacDonald repeated his arguments of the previous evening. The White House, he explained, "didn't disagree with the goals [of the report]; we disagreed with the implementations."

As spokesman for the Commission, Judy Woodruff introduced Dr. Beny J. Primm, the single black on the Commission and its specialist on drug abuse. "Dr. Primm," said Woodruff, "you were quoted yesterday as saying that you were shocked at the White House's response [to the report]. Why was that?"

Overnight, apparently, Dr. Primm had had second thoughts. Of his outburst the previous day, Dr. Primm declared: "I talked about it from a different perspective. . . . Despite the fact that [the president] did not endorse that particular segment [the proposal for a federal law against discrimination], the work will be done by the . . . Office of Personnel Management."

Reassured by MacDonald's assent, Primm yielded a step further. "If this thing gets to the attorney-general and gets back to the president in an expeditious manner, then there's no question that . . . anti-discrimination should become a law." Further apologizing for his sharp criticism of the previous day, Primm declared: "I think that what we need to do here is to look at our biases that give us different perceptions of what people say and what people write. Certainly my bias would be to have $1.6 billion in place per year for the next two years . . . to start 2,500 new drug treatment programs. . . . However, if this money is phased in over time, and we get up to that amount so that treatment is available to all who need it, I will be satisfied."

Gratified by Primm's newly discovered prudence, MacDonald assured him and

---

[1] In June 1988, before the publication of the Commission's Final Report, Admiral Watkins had, indeed, proposed the appointment of what the media denominated as "an AIDS czar," a single official to promote "expeditious movement, more collaboration, shared reagents—someone to integrate, coordinate actions within a national plan." The surgeon general, Watkins suggested, "could bring an end to the bureaucratic anarchy if granted special authority by the President for some years and empowered to replace the Office of Management and Budget in supervision of FDA and NIH research efforts." Watkins said he had had "to back off [on this proposal] to get consensus [among the commissioners] on our final report."

Asked by Ted Koppel of ABC's "Nightline" for his response to Watkins's suggestion, Surgeon General Koop replied: "I think what you really need within our department is a way of facilitating the getting of the things that are essential to move ahead so that the bureaucratic barriers that we all understand quite well are removed. Somebody who had that kind of power would add a great deal to this whole battle. If offered the job, I'd certainly have to consider it."

the audience that "the president clearly is strongly opposed to drug abuse and has put a strong package."

Primm was determined to make clear his total conversion. "I think," he declared, repeating an argument MacDonald had been using,

> that when we get a clear explanation of what the thought was behind each one of these 10 [presidential] recommendations . . . we will see that we are more in concurrence with one another than in incongruence. . . . the hue and cry now is that we need leadership from the highest point. . . . The president is extremely supportive, as far as I am concerned, is extremely concerned about this issue. I am more hopeful now than I was yesterday. Maybe I reacted yesterday a bit too zealously because I brought my own biases to this issue.

What had happened overnight to Dr. Primm?

As for the czar proclaimed by Dr. MacDonald—President Reagan—what had he accomplished against the epidemic during the previous six years?

The Presidential Candidates and the Report

On June 28, the day after the transmission of the Final Report to the president, staff members of the Presidential Commission were elated at expressions of approval by both 1988 presidential candidates. In fact, however, their exuberance seemed rather to expose a low level of expectations than justified satisfaction.

On June 24 Michael Dukakis's office issued a statement congratulating "Admiral Watkins and the members of the Presidential Commission on AIDS for their comprehensive and insightful report on the HIV epidemic." The press release expressed support for proposals in the Report for tougher antidiscrimination and confidentiality measures, for expanded education and research programs and for innovative approaches to providing care. It expressed the hope "that the President [would] be encouraged by this report to put together a national plan to guide us in a war on AIDS. . . . his generals in this war must be public health officials, not OMB budget analysts." The statement called for "accelerated drug treatment trials and research efforts."

If the statement, undoubtedly drafted by public relations personnel, left little to be desired by the Commission, in subsequent campaign statements, Dukakis avoided all mention of the AIDS crisis.

On June 29, the *New York Times* noted that "in contrast to President Reagan, Vice President Bush today quickly endorsed legislation and other Federal measures that would prohibit discrimination against AIDS victims . . . [and] said he supported the issuing of a Presidential order to put in place voluntary guidelines barring discrimination against AIDS victims in the Federal workplace and Federal legislation outlawing the practice elsewhere." Mr. Bush framed his discussion of the report (which he admitted he had not read) in terms of the disease's effect on children. "My conscience has been advising me on AIDS," the paper quoted Bush as saying. "I'd hate it if a kid of mine got a blood transfusion and my grandson had AIDS and the community discriminated against the child, that innocent child." For gays and IV drug users, presumably, Mr. Bush had little concern. Asked why the president had not responded to the report as quickly as he, the vice president quipped, "Well, he's not running for president."

According to *New York Newsday* on August 14, when Senator Lowell Weicker urged the Republican Platform Committee to endorse the Commission's recommendations on an antidiscrimination and confidentiality law, "Bush, who has parted company with Reagan in supporting affirmative action and laws prohibiting discrimination against those who have AIDS, did not fight for those positions in the Republican platform, and the more conservative views prevailed." A Bush aide questioned by the *Newsday* reporter said she could not explain the paradox.

Furthermore, while publicly declaring his support for antidiscrimination legislation, according to the *Washington Post* of June 29, 1988, "Bush told reporters he did not favor an immediate increase in federal research funds because Dr. Anthony S. Fauci of the National Institutes of Health told him at a dinner at his home two nights ago that the funding allocated to NIH for that purpose now is about 'right.'"

That assurance to the presidential candidate ran counter to Fauci's testimony little more than two months earlier before the Weiss House subcommittee, when Fauci had admitted that his Institute was critically hampered in its functions by a shortage of staff and lack of adequate office and laboratory space. At best Fauci was being disingenuous. Even if he had subsequently decided that he had received sufficient additions to his staff, could it be that he as a director of the NIH AIDS program was unaware that additional research funds were needed for clinical trials throughout the nation as well as for AIDS research at CDC and FDA? How could he, in good conscience, reject so cavalierly the incontrovertible evidence to the contrary in the Commission's Final Report?

Fauci, apparently, was still telling superiors what he thought they wanted to hear.

Confident of Fauci's certain support even of the cut in AIDS appropriations he was planning, Bush hastened to express his gratitude. Asked at a presidential candidates' debate whom he would list as heroes in the contemporary United States, Bush picked Fauci as his first choice.

◆ ◆ ◆

A day after the publication of the president's response to the Final Report, Bush asked Dr. Young "as quickly as possible" to develop "new [FDA] administrative and legislative proposals" to speed the availability of new drugs for life-threatening conditions that lack adequate therapies. "The effort to help dying patients, together with the emphasis placed on Mr. Bush's role," the *New York Times* commented, "could distance his Presidential campaign from the criticism of a lack of presidential leadership." Prodded by a Cabinet-level study group headed by Bush, FDA, according to the *Times*, "started quietly last Monday to re-examine virtually all stages of the long process by which drugs for such [life-threatening] diseases are now tested and approved for marketing."

The *Times* cited unnamed officials as saying that "the proposed changes would almost certainly produce faster decisions. But whether they would produce many more useful drugs [was] problematic. The result for most experimental drugs could be faster rejection, not faster approval." One official, "who requested that his name be withheld," added, "You're not going to change the rules and all of a sudden spring loose a zillion drugs for AIDS."

On September 7, 1988 the *New York Times* reported a difference in attitude between the two presidential candidates: Michael Dukakis, following the direction in the Final Report, favored expansion of the drug treatment programs to guarantee treatment to any intravenous drug user who sought help; George Bush, stressing "harsher penalties . . . ha[d] not focused on treatment of addiction."

Indeed, despite the flurry of electioneering rhetoric, it would be up to the Congress to implement the recommendations of the president's AIDS Commission. On September 7 the *New York Times* reported that in a change of strategy from emphasizing the halt of the supply of drugs to an emphasis on treatment of drug addiction, a change "influenced by the report of the Presidential Commission on AIDS, which tied intravenous drug use to AIDS and to crime," a $2 billion drug bill was expected to receive bipartisan support in the House, and maneuvering was under way to pass a similar bill in the Senate. The Congress recognized that "if enough treatment were available, tens or hundreds of thousands of lives could be saved."

Senator Alan Cranston amended the Labor–HHS appropriations act to require the NIH to "take all possible steps to ensure that eleven experimental drugs for the treatment of AIDS that [had] shown some effectiveness [were] tested in clinical trials as expeditiously as possible and with as many subjects as are scientifically acceptable"; and Congress voted to establish a new national AIDS commission to implement the Watkins's Commission's recommendations. In addition, Congress appropriated $5 million in support of community research groups like the New York Consumer Research Initiative.

◆ ◆ ◆

In his budget message to Congress on February 8, 1989, after speaking of "the terrible tragedy of AIDS," President Bush requested an appropriation $300 million less for AIDS services than the request submitted by Reagan's Department of Health and Human Services.

Two weeks later, however, at hearings of the House Subcommittee on Human Resources, a "new" Anthony Fauci, newly appointed adviser to President Bush on AIDS matters, urged greater flexibility from FDA in releasing emergency AIDS therapies. Questioning by the subcommittee revealed, however, that Bush and his associates were more prepared to berate FDA than to provide it with additional funds. Similarly, the administration cut a Centers for Disease Control request for $116 million to combat AIDS in minority communities to a mere $16.5 million and gutted a request for dealing with the spread of AIDS among drug abusers. Commented Congressman Donald Paine, who represented an AIDS-devastated district in Newark, New Jersey: "This seems to me to be a very passive attitude to take when we have a volcano erupting."

◆ ◆ ◆

In the spring of 1988, Admiral Watkins wrote a letter to the Class of 1992 at the Naval Academy in which he reminded the cadets of their particular responsibility to the nation: "Society expects you to be on top of things, they expect you to follow ethical practices, they expect you to be the paragon of excellence. . . . They need you as a benchmark for excellence."

In explanation of this letter, Admiral Watkins declared: "We have decided that this is a self-indulgent, permissive society. We've built it that way. The old approach of assimilating a national tradition of the Declaration of Independence and the Gettysburg Address has been maligned. Instead, we inculcate in people a spirit that is really anti-freedom. We've got to recognize that that is not a very smart idea. We've got to go back and fix it. That's going to take a long time."

Questioned as to how he would evaluate expenditures for the military, the major emphasis of Reagan policy, as against funds to combat the AIDS epidemic, the former Chief of Naval Operations responded without equivocation:

I . . . believe they [national security and the AIDS crisis] are closely connected. It's not just AIDS and national security. . . . We have given short shrift to the readiness of the nation's human resources, readiness in the work place, readiness to compete, readiness to survive in our society. . . . The military today is more competitive than the private sector because they've got an assured salary, assured job, exciting work, new equipment. . . . But . . . the national security has been weakened because private sector resources are inadequate. My feeling is that we have at the heart of this HIV the evidence that the human resources of this nation are so important to national security that you better define the AIDS crisis as such and make it an element of national security and quit trying to pair off one against the other.

With the termination of his chairmanship, the Admiral was eager to proceed to new endeavors. "I'm now a zealot," he said.

The AIDS investigation has given me additional adrenalin. It exposed the villains in our society. . . .

I'm going to stay in the fight, but not on the AIDS issue, I'm going to stay for the larger issue. If you look at the long-term education proposals in our Report where I harp on the social context of the AIDS crisis, you will see that my personal bias is that if we go AIDS specific, if we go substance abuse specific, pregnancy specific, nutrition specific—all those band aids—we don't know what the hell we're doing. . . . I have very deep feelings about this epidemic as having the potential to be a very powerful catalyst for major restructuring of our thinking in the country—in the schools, health care delivery, you name it.

Asked what hope he had of significant leadership from either of the presidential candidates in the resolution of the national crises, Admiral Watkins was not optimistic. "I don't see that happening with either candidate. I don't see the broader vision. It's going to be, throw more money at standby programs that haven't done well in the past, but it's not going to be an attack on the fundamental problems."

On January 11, 1989 President-elect George Bush announced the appointment of Admiral James D. Watkins (ret.) as Secretary of Energy. If in his new position Admiral Watkins would no longer exert influence in the implementation of the recommendations of the Commission he had recently headed, the war against AIDS would suffer the loss of an important spokesman and dedicated fighter.

Aftermath

"We don't have a Federal policy on AIDS, period."

"Having missed the opportunity to get the ounce of prevention, we now have to pay for pounds and pounds of cure."

So spoke, respectively, former U.S. Surgeon General C. Everett Koop and Representative Henry A. Waxman before the House Subcommittee on Health and the Environment on February 27, 1989.

Two years later several leaders of the AIDS community who had served as expert witnesses for the Presidential Commission were asked to respond to two questions: (1) What do you consider the most significant changes in the struggle during the last two years? and (2) What are the major issues and problems confronting the AIDS community a year and a half after the appearance of the Final Report of the Presidential Commission?

Dr. Stephen Nicholas

Dr. Stephen Nicholas[1] was not only dividing his time as a pediatrician between Columbia Presbyterian and Harlem Hospital but was in attendance at Incarnation Children's Center as well, with some eighty HIV-infected children under his supervision. In planning two years earlier, the center was now in full operation as a residence for infected children abandoned in hospitals. One hundred and forty-seven children from various New York institutions had passed through its doors, of whom 123 had been placed in foster homes after an average stay of from forty days to two months (an average skewed by the longer stay of the sickest children).

---

[1] Stephen Nicholas was interviewed during the summer of 1988. See pp. 127–132 in Chapter 12.

A major change in the struggle against the AIDS epidemic during the previous two years, according to Nicholas, had developed out of an increasing recognition of HIV infection among women and children. Nicholas was convinced that publicity about the little boy adopted at birth by the hospital staff whose delightful personality profoundly moved Admiral Watkins during his visit to the hospital helped to promote this recognition. (The child died just before reaching his fourth birthday.)

An ongoing study of some 400 pregnant women with HIV infection begun four years ago in four city hospitals—a study in which Nicholas was participating—seemed to point to about a 30 percent transmission of the virus to offspring.

According to Nicholas advances were being made in earlier diagnosis of HIV infection among infants. He anticipated that in the near future infection would be detected among asymptomatic infants within six months although twelve to fifteen months would still be required to determine whether infants of infected mothers were free of infection. In addition, the authorization of AZT for children infected with the virus made it more likely that children would live longer. "We now have children," he said, "who have reached the age of 11."

Another major change, Nicholas asserted, was the loss of fear and an increase in compassion for HIV-infected infants, and he was gratified by the number of people who were coming forward to serve as foster parents, mostly black and Hispanic—a larger percentage middle-class than among the general roster of foster parents. In addition, a sizable number of single men, many openly gay, were accepting the children into their homes.

How would Nicholas characterize these volunteer foster parents?

"Saintly."

Frustrated by the lack of communication among groups providing services to HIV patients, Nicholas had instituted a course open to first-year medical, nursing, and social work students on the medical and social problems in pediatric AIDS, a course probably unique in the nation. Members of his class developed friendships, he said, which he hoped would continue through their careers to the benefit of the HIV-infected people with whom they would be working.

Nicholas was encouraged by the fact that the number of cases among infants in New York City appeared to have reached a plateau with no significant spread of the infection among middle-class women. Nevertheless, such an expansion, he warned, might still occur. As yet to be confronted, he said, were the critical social ramifications arising from the fact that AIDS among women and children remained primarily a disease of the poor.

Iris Long, Ph.D., and Iris L. Davis, M.D.

Beginning her AIDS volunteer work in 1986 on the GMHC hotline, Dr. Iris Long became acquainted with the varied ramifications of HIV infection. With the establishment of the Community Research Initiative she assumed responsibility for the development of community research projects among local physicians with extensive

AIDS practices. Upon the formation of ACT UP Long undertook a leading role on the organization's Issues Committee and on the data section of the Treatment and Data Subcommittee. Her activities brought her into contact with FDA, NIH and state and municipal AIDS agencies, and she was invited to testify before Congressional committees and the Presidential Commission.

From 1988 to 1990 Long issued six "AIDS Treatment Registry Reports" on AIDS clinical trials. A paper entitled "Demographic Analysis of ACTU Trial Enrollment vs. Incidence of AIDS in New York City," which she read at the VIth International Conference on AIDS in San Francisco in June 1990 was praised as a major contribution in the field.

"Now we have the data," Dr. Long declared. "We know that the segments of the population which are currently most endangered by HIV infection are receiving least attention: children and their families, women, IV drug abusers and prisoners. These groups are composed primarily of the minorities, people with the least voice and power in the society. The leadership of their struggle must come from within the communities."

Dr. Iris Davis, who had transferred from her position as supervisor of the AIDS program at Woodhull Hospital in Brooklyn to a post at Cornell University's New York Hospital,[2] blamed the failure of the established AIDS activist organizations to reach out to the minorities on the lack of cultural sophistication and class prejudice pervading American society.

Late in 1989, Iris Long, Iris Davis and other activists organized AIDS Treatment Resources (ATR), an informal and unaffiliated committee directed toward building coalitions within the endangered and neglected populations. In June 1990, with funding from the New York State Department of Health AIDS Institute, ATR published a mammoth 420-page study entitled "Access to AIDS Clinical Trials and Experimental Drugs in New York State." After conducting "interviews with trial site staff and collecting demographic and epidemiologic data from federal, state and city AIDS surveillance groups," the investigators arrived at two major conclusions: "that clinical research in New York State occurs without systematic coordination, oversight, planning or outreach; and that many potential trial participants are excluded due to lack of access to health care, researcher bias and poor trial design."[3]

In its detail and comprehensiveness, the ATR report exemplified the expertise and broad experience of its drafters. The report covered much of the same ground as the 1988 "Final Report of the Presidential Commission on the HIV Infection"

---

[2] Dr. Davis was interviewed during the summer of 1988. See pp. 132–135 in Chapter 12.

[3] According to the New York State Department of Health, as of January 31, 1990, 85.7 percent of the people diagnosed with AIDS in the state were male and 14.3 percent (33 percent of the national total) were female; 38.2 percent white, 34.4 percent black, and 26.1 percent Hispanic—or, respectively, 15.8 percent, 29.0 percent, and 38.7 percent of the PWAs in the nation who come from these groups. People with a history of IV drug use accounted for 42.6 percent (34.9 percent of the national total of the state AIDS caseload with a conservative estimate of 120,000 or more IV drug users infected with HIV in New York City).

and revealed that the critical problems of funding; staffing; facilities; bureaucratic overlapping; wasteful interagency competition; lack of coordination among federal, state and municipal agencies; and failure to disseminate information widely and quickly had not been effectively addressed in the two years since the publication of the Commission's report. The ATR report also criticized the secrecy regarding results of research and evaluations of clinical trials and noted the absence of input by local AIDS communities and health care providers and the concomitant domination of AIDS research by "a small number of investigators with limited clinical trial experience" who were failing "to entertain dissenting scientific views and conflicts of authority among committees dealing with the epidemic."

The investigation revealed that Medicaid recipients were seriously underrepresented in clinical trials, that prisoners with AIDS in state correctional facilities—constituting 25 percent of the AIDS population in New York State outside New York City—received severely inadequate health care, that support services for people with AIDS and HIV infection were severely lacking and that "a major factor in lack of appropriate primary care provision [was] lack of information" among both people with AIDS/HIV and health care practitioners.

For a large proportion of people infected with HIV, the report noted, only enrolment in a clinical trial guaranteed consistent supervision and treatment. Nevertheless, of a total of 121,645 cases of AIDS reported in the United States through January 31, 1990 (with an estimated 49,067 still living, or 40.3 percent of the total), "9,505 patients, both adults and children," the report declared, "have been enrolled in 102 ACTG clinical trials . . . 7.8% of the national AIDS caseload. . . . The majority of states," the report went on to state, "have fewer than three trials currently enrolling. Patients in these locales have only a slim chance of finding a trial which meets their needs and for which they are eligible."

The report expressed sharp criticism in an area skirted by the Presidential Commission. "In an epidemic," the report warned, "competitiveness hinders expedient development of AIDS drugs. Federal legislation should state that when public health concerns clash with a drug company's claim of proprietary rights, the issue must be decided in favor of the public health." As for research by drug companies, the report declared, "the main concern is profit, not health care. . . . priorities are decided by business people, not by research scientists and certainly not by community members."

"The ACTG," the report went on to recommend, "should standardize procedures for providing everyone who is eligible for a trial with health care. . . . Of course, national legislation that recognizes universal health care as a citizen's right and commits the resources to help citizens secure this right would eliminate the problem."

For a November 1990 conference in Washington, D.C. on Access in Experimental Treatments, Drs. Long and Davis prepared a paper entitled "New York Women in Aids Clinical Trials" in which they pointed out that "by 1989 HIV/AIDS death rates among New York and New Jersey African-American women between the ages of 15 and 44 were comparable to those among adult women in Abidjan, the capital city . . . of the Ivory Coast . . . [and that] studies predict[ed] continuously escalating death rates among women of childbearing age." They cited a prognosis in a study conducted at the Montefiore Medical Center in the Bronx that during the last five years of the century "30,000 to 40,000 African-American and Latino children in the New York City . . . area [would] have lost both parents to AIDS." In their paper the two women noted complaints of black leaders that they were subject to disrespect from some ACT UP members. "When Black leaders have attempted to educate themselves about homosexuality and to overcome homophobic attitudes," they asserted, "it is time for Lesbian and gay AIDS activists to take stock of their scornful and stereotypical attitudes toward Black medical, public health, political and community leaders."

Speaking out of her hospital experience, Dr. Davis noted that with the expansion of the infection among the minorities and the poor the health services were strained ever more acutely and that funds were not being provided to meet the growing crisis. On the other hand, she was encouraged by the fact that black churches and established organizations were overcoming their homophobia and addressing the threat of the epidemic in their community. Activist organizations, she noted, were springing up in black communities throughout the nation (more slowly in the Hispanic community). A national association of beauty parlors, she noted, had undertaken to conduct an educational campaign among their clients. She herself had become more dedicated in the struggle to educate and mobilize the unempowered population, devoting more and more of her energies in addressing groups in the black and Hispanic communities and expressing her views as a member of a subcommittee of the ACTG as well as at various other AIDS committees.

Bill Bahlman

A year and a half after terminating his role as ACT UP watchdog with the Presidential Commission, Bill Bahlman continued to attend conferences. He presented a paper at the Vth International Conference on AIDS in Montreal in June 1988 entitled "AIDS Activism: A Means for Productive Change to Promote Clinical Research and Drug Development." He was participating in the gay and lesbian weekly hour on Public Access cable television, presenting videotapes he took of demonstrations, interviewing personalities like Anthony Fauci of NIAID and conducting a series called "Bill Bahlman's hit list," in which he exposed people with homophobic agendas or people blocking the progress in the campaign against the virus.

Diagnosed as HIV-positive in January 1989, late in 1990 Bahlman enrolled in an ACTG intramural trial of a new, as yet unnamed drug that in in vitro tests had revealed far greater potency than AZT. "Up to now," he noted, "the emphasis has been on development of anti-virals, which prolong life for greater or lesser periods of time. Now development of treatments to reconstitute immunity is necessary to prevent premature death of those infected with HIV."

Bahlman was encouraged by the acceleration of the approval process of HIV therapies, by the increasing access to clinical trials for previously neglected elements of the population and by the development of a parallel track under which PWAs who failed to respond to approved therapies could be treated by promising but as yet unapproved therapies. Indeed, he declared, the ACT UP agenda developed in 1987 and 1988 had for the most part been adopted as official policy.

Regarding research, testing and authorization of AIDS therapies, in his year-end statement in the December 21, 1990 *AIDS Treatment News*, John James, too, expressed restrained optimism. He observed an unprecedented interest in changing "policies and procedures which made the sacrifice of part of a generation inevitable." He warned, however, of continuing major problems in delays in treatment development "especially in the often-secret preclinical phase and sometimes in the U.S. Patent Office. . . . Research funding," he insisted, was "becoming more critical as money [was] taken away from research to pay for AZT or other patient care. Congressional advocacy for treatment access had barely begun. To avoid major unnecessary delays and obstacles," he warned, "community intelligence, communication, coalition and pressure must continue."

The 1991 Report of the Follow-up National Commission

In September 1991 the National Commission on Acquired Immune Deficiency Syndrome appointed by President Bush two years earlier to monitor the responses to the recommendations of the 1988 Final Report of the Watkins Commission issued its own 165-page report, "Americans Living with AIDS." A quotation on the cover from one of the thousand or so witnesses testifying before this new commission sets the tone: "I ask that this Commission take back to Washington and to the President my voice of hope for the future and discontent with the past." The motto on the title page conveys the impatience and dismay of the Commission itself: "Transforming Anger, Fear, and Indifference into Action." The leitmotif throughout the document echoes that of the Watkins report: "Articulate leadership guiding Americans toward a proper response to AIDS has been notably absent."

In its recommendations, the new commission, under its competent and principled chairperson June E. Osborn, M.D., professor of epidemiology and dean of the School of Public Health of the University of Michigan, gave evidence that the recommendations of the preceding Commission had simply been shelved by the Bush administration. The new commission repeated the recommendation for the establishment of a "comprehensive national HIV plan," noting that one-third of the 100,000 deaths from AIDS had occurred in the single year of 1990, an increasing percentage of these outside the previous centers of the epidemic and previously affected population segments. By 1993 the report projected a rise in the number of cases to over 350,000 with "AIDS clearly outstrip[ping] all other diseases in lost human potential." The new commission renewed the recommendations of its predecessor in regard to funding for research and treatment, broader participation of underrepresented populations in clinical trials, increased training programs for health care providers, more effective dissemination of treatment information, evaluation of antidiscrimination laws at all levels of government, broader access to drugs and increased support of community-based organizations.

(This latter appeal arrived too late for the Community Research Initiative, the New York City effort launched with so much promise in 1986. Unable to meet its rent and other expenses, CRI was dissolved in October 1991.)

From its travels and hearings throughout the nation, the Osborn Commission, like the Watkins Commission, concluded "that HIV disease could not be understood outside the context of racism, homophobia, poverty and unemployment."

Abandoning the caution of the Watkins Commission and in defiance of the administration that had appointed it, the Osborn Commission proclaimed: "Our nation must do what virtually every other major industrialized nation has done— adopt a universal health plan that ensures access to health care for all its citizens." It called treatment of all IVDUs who request it "a matter of national urgency" and decried the moralistic opposition to frank sex education as well as the "withholding of potentially lifesaving information and devices in order to avoid a public presumed to be in agreement with such constraints."

With the Bush administration like its predecessor exhibiting apathy and indifference in the face of the national crisis, the AIDS community would have to continue to provide leadership and to exert unrelenting pressure in order to assure that even minimal measures were pursued against the HIV scourge.

the five principal opportunistic infections treatable or preventable within eighteen months. Representatives of FDA and NIH, of pharmaceutical companies and of the Congress were invited to a discussion of the new program, and a twenty-five-page booklet was distributed with detailed proposals for its implementation. "Countdown" represented a major achievement for ACT UP New York and gave evidence of the maturity, unflagging militancy and imagination in the activist movement.

A month later, responding to pressure from the women's caucus of ACT UP, Fauci convened the first National Conference on Women and HIV Infection.

Iris Long, an activist with a five-year history of devoted participation and a leader in its treatment and data programs, looked back with pride at the achievements of ACT UP. "Beginning without any organizational experience," she declared,

> we mobilized, we learned where and how to struggle and made important contributions in data gathering and in promoting research and clinical testing. We brought pressure upon FDA and NIH to expand clinical testing, to publicize research and clinical tests and to broaden participation in tests. Because of our pressure, rules and regulations have been modified, and FDA and NIH have been empowered to accelerate research activities and approval of new therapies.

Another activist of many years, deeply involved in the general evolution and day-by-day activities of ACT UP, Suzanne Philipps (an intern at the time of her introduction in this book at the meeting in February 1987 at which Michael May reported his extraordinary improvement after treatment with AL721), was more restrained in her evaluation of the organization's history:

> Years ago, when we met at the lesbian and gay community center, we were standing shoulder to shoulder in a large family gathering. After the well-publicized action at St. Patrick's Cathedral in December 1988, the membership expanded abruptly beyond the initial white and middle-class founders. Caucuses of Asian and Pacific Islanders, Latinos-Latinas and Afro-Americans were organized [the latter caucus the weakest because of unresolved problems with the general community], and at meetings ten to fifteen per cent of those in attendance were people of color.

With the increasing awareness of the broad social and political ramifications of the struggle, Suzanne Philipps noted, committees focusing on special issues sprang up—on homelessness, women and children with HIV infection, prisoners infected with the virus, the collapsing national health service and even "Against the New World Order."

With the new, expanded approach the organization confronted a risk of being overwhelmed by involvement in numerous complex, long-range and seemingly intractable problems. Difficulties arose, too, from adventurism and an anarchistic resistance to centralized administration among a portion of the membership. In adapting to new circumstances, Philipps stated, older members proved a stabilizing force. "Some months ago," she declared, we managed to persuade the membership to empower a coordinating committee composed primarily of representatives of the various committees to set the agenda and to select priorities. We are learning to distinguish between what must be taken care of tonight and what can wait until next week.

We are at a crucial point in our history and have to be realistic. We came to ACT UP with fire in our hearts and with a conviction that if we fought long and hard enough and loved each other enough, we would slay the Medusa. Now we walk on a psychological tightrope, more than ever conscious that we live under the sword of Damocles.

Nevertheless, she added, "I can't imagine that ACT UP will ever die. It is so important for the AIDS community in providing fellowship, support and a focus for activity and exchange of information. We have, in addition, the responsibility of bearing witness so that our history and our accomplishments will not be forgotten."

The achievements in the AIDS war were not won without casualties among hundreds of dedicated and courageous activists like Tom Hannan of New York, Jim Sammone of Orlando and John Fox and Tom O'Connor of San Francisco.

On May 29, 1989, after months of deterioration, Barry Gingell, medical consultant for GMHC, died. At a memorial service at St. Peter's Episcopal Church on June 24 three of his closest associates described how Barry had enriched their lives, added strength to the AIDS community and devoted his last energies to helping others suffering from the viral infection. In his numerous interventions before various committees and before the Presidential Commission, Barry had cut through the obfuscations of officials of FDA and NIH and exposed the full scope of the epidemic and the bureaucratic failure to confront the crisis head-on.

Said AIDS lawyer Jay Lipner in his eulogy: "When asked whom he would name as contemporary American heroes, then presidential candidate George Bush named Anthony Fauci first of all. We in the AIDS community," said Lipner, "without question choose Barry Gingell."[1]

Many other "winter soldiers" never extolled by the media or in the AIDS community sacrificed their time and energy and even their lives in the struggle. Among these heroes are the dozens of physicians, gay and straight, who treated the infected throughout the nation. One such was Stuart, son of lawyer Arnold Forster who offered assistance to the New York activists at the first distribution of AL721 in April 1987. After his death in February 1991 from a heart attack at age 44, Stubsy, as he was known to his friends and patients, was eulogized in the gay publication "Outweek" by the surviving partner of one of Stubsy's patients:

From the beginning of the epidemic, Stubsy . . . rejected any notion that a health professional should avoid patients with AIDS. He provided care to middle class gay men, to poor IV-drug users and to anyone else who needed

---

[1] On October 18, 1989 the Department of Health and Human Services presented a posthumous award to Dr. Barry Gingell.

it . . . the best care possible—even that put him in conflict with the medical establishment. . . . Stubsy's personal caring went beyond that of "bedside manner." Each patient was an individual treated with respect and affection. . . . He fought unstintingly for his patients' lives, for their rights and for their dignity. . . . he exemplified a professionalism free of homophobia. . . . He was one of our bravest friends.

Perhaps the greatest contribution of the AIDS community to the nation and to the American democratic heritage lay in the example it provided of the power that could be mobilized by a minority in defense of their rights and their very lives. Grudgingly the Reagan administration was compelled to listen. The general population watched with growing respect, and even the Moral Majority grew more cautious in its vilification.

As early as 1987 the Lavender Hill Mob had demonstrated an awareness that the AIDS crisis could not be dissociated from problems of homophobia, racism, illiteracy and poverty. In recognition of the broader implications of the struggle, two Mobsters appeared at a CDC conference in the garb of Nazi concentration camp inmates. Recognizing the links between homophobia and racism, the Mob participated in a demonstration protesting the Howard Beach attacks on three black men. In a leaflet entitled "AIDS: Politics and Prejudice," the Mob associated the government's failure to confront the spread of AIDS in the minority communities with questions of military and foreign policy, noting:

> The Pentagon spends more money in just one day than the Federal government has spent on AIDS research in seven years. It is expected that more Americans will die of AIDS than died in the entire Vietnam war.

By late 1990, with ever more alarming estimates regarding the spread of the epidemic and with declining hope of the inauguration of the Manhattan Project against AIDS that Michael Callen called for before the Presidential Commission, the entire gay activist community had advanced to a recognition that the struggle would continue indefinitely, ever requiring new strategies and tactics on a broader battle front.

When the AIDS crisis is set within the context of the many other crises threatening the nation—the destruction of the environment, the collapse of the health care service system, the bankruptcy of the educational system, the expansion of the underclass and the widening gap between rich and poor along with the uncertainty of the national and world economies—then it becomes apparent that the very survival of American democracy may be at stake. Under this view, the AIDS crisis represents a grim symptom of a pervasive and more profound malaise. Grappling with the ramifications of the AIDS crisis, in effect, serves as a testing of America, that is, of the nation's will to mount the kind of effort mobilized by the AIDS community against the virus for a restoration of the entire commonwealth.

As a result of his experiences as chairman of the Presidential Commission on the HIV epidemic, Admiral Watkins became convinced that a massive national effort was required to deal not just with the AIDS epidemic but with the general social, political and economic crisis in the United States. On July 20, 1988 he declared:

> If this nation really decided to have an America 2000 movement, and we were going to get the human resources literate, healthy and motivated to the job, get the kids back in school, get them in the mainstream, give them not only the incentive but a sure job . . . if we got the people motivated to . . . make service to others a good thing again in our society—we would do more for national security than a couple of carrier battle groups, a division of the army in Europe. . . . If you're going to agree to restructure the nation, then restructure it in transition to a better America that has a stronger, more motivated democratic concept so imbued in our people that they really believe it.

How great was the possibility for such a 2000 movement?

> If we wanted to make this AIDS crisis the Pearl Harbor of our human resources as a nation, really mobilize for it in its broadest context of improved education for our young people, of improved education in the workplace, a greater love for each other, a greater understanding of the cultures that make up our society, everyone pulling together—in twelve years you'd have a nation that is so far ahead of everybody else in the world, you'd have 50 years in which you could probably just live on it, ride the bow wave. . . . The probability is small, the possibilities are tremendous.

Four years after the publication of the Final Report of the Watkins Commission, as Drs. Nicholas, Long and Davis emphasized and as the report of the follow-up Osborn Commission evidenced, the nation had still not begun to confront the social problems providing the environment for the spread of the epidemic, and an "America 2000 movement" for restructuring the United States in a transition to a kinder and truly more secure nation seemed no more likely of realization than when Admiral Watkins proposed it.

Would the nation have to confront crises even more menacing before it recognized the need for the major restructuring of American society?

INDEX

◆ ◆ ◆

229

DATE DUE